# THE

DATE DUE

# GOLD'S GYM

# GUIDE TO GETTING
# STARTED
# IN BODY
# BUILDING

## THE AUTHORITY ON FITNESS SINCE 1965

### ED HOUSEWRIGHT

**McGraw-Hill**

New York   Chicago   San Francisco   Lisbon   London   Madrid   Mexico City
Milan   New Delhi   San Juan   Seoul   Singapore   Sydney   Toronto

The McGraw·Hill Companies

**Library of Congress Cataloging-in-Publication Data**

Housewright, Ed.
    The Official Gold's Gym Guide to Getting Started in Bodybuilding / by Ed Housewright.
        p.   cm.
    Includes bibliographical references (p.      ) and index.
    ISBN 0-07-142284-6

    1. Bodybuilding—Handbooks, manuals, etc.  I. Title: Guide to getting started
    in bodybuilding.  II. Gold's Gym.  III. Title.

    GV546.5.H68  2005
    613.7'13—dc22                                                    2004008276

1 2 3 4 5 6 7 8 9 0   QPD/QPD   3 2 1 0 9 8 7 6 5 4

ISBN 0-07-142284-6

This book is printed on acid-free paper.

To my parents,
who have supported me in everything I've done,
and my son,
who has brought me indescribable joy

# CONTENTS

# ACKNOWLEDGMENTS

This book was developed and produced by Mountain Lion, Inc., a book producer specializing in fitness, sports, and general reference books. A book producer relies on the special skills of many people. The following contributed to producing this book; to all of them we say "thanks."

- Mark Weinstein, editor at McGraw-Hill Trade, whose guidance and suggestions were instrumental in moving this project through its various stages
- Ed Powderly, Senior Vice President of Product Licensing of Gold's Gym International, who contributed significantly to formulating the book's overall content, including the editorial scope and photographic treatment
- Maureen Babcock of Gold's Gym, who gathered and sent us the appropriate Gold's Gym apparel for our fitness demonstrators
- Ken Strickland, former U.S. Marine Corps Sergeant Major and manager of the Gold's Gym located on the outskirts of Princeton, New Jersey, who arranged and coordinated our photography sessions (Ken runs his gym facility with an exemplary *esprit de corps,* pursuing his fitness mission with an infectious enthusiasm.)
- Randy and Bonnie Vey, owners and operators of the spectacular and award-winning Princeton Gold's Gym facility, and their staff
- John Monteleone and Vicki Russo at Mountain Lion, Inc., who shepherded the project from concept to finished manuscript and completed photographs
- Ed Housewright, who researched and wrote the text
- Barry Havens, photographer, who expertly handled all the photography
- Avery Stephenson and Mike Martin, our Gold's Stars, who ably demonstrated the exercises in all of the beginner bodybuilding workout programs

Bodybuilding has come a long way. Just look at photos of champion bodybuilders in the 1940s or '50s and compare them to today's champs.

There is no comparison. Today's top bodybuilders boast muscles that are far bigger, better defined, and more symmetrical than those of their counterparts just a few decades ago.

In many ways, this is the golden age of bodybuilding. Advances in training techniques and nutrition have made it possible for more people to achieve a rock-hard physique that once seemed out of reach. Granted, building a great body isn't simple. It still takes dedication, persistence, and patience, but today there's a road map—a set of proven training principles—to help you on your journey.

Bodybuilding stars of the past, including the famous Arnold Schwarzenegger, often had to rely on trial and error to make gains. They experimented with a range of training methods and nutritional approaches, never quite sure what would work for them. Today, beginning bodybuilders can benefit from the lessons of their predecessors and make far greater gains in far less time.

*The Official Gold's Gym Guide to Getting Started in Bodybuilding* will teach you to awaken your dormant muscles and transform your physique, using the latest knowledge and most advanced techniques. Gold's Gym has been the undisputed leader in bodybuilding for almost 40 years, dating back to the opening of the original Gold's Gym in Venice, California, in 1965. That now-famous gym became the mecca for the world's top bodybuilders in the 1960s and '70s. It provided the backdrop for the 1976 movie *Pumping Iron,* which opened up the world of bodybuilding to the public. Today, Gold's has more than 500 gyms worldwide. There's probably one near your home.

Let's be clear. We don't promise overnight miracles. *The Official Gold's Gym Guide to Getting Started in Bodybuilding* won't turn a 98-pound weakling or a flabby couch potato into a world champion bodybuilder in 30 days, as some books and products seem to promise. We'll leave the grandiose, unrealistic claims to others.

Instead, *The Official Gold's Gym Guide to Getting Started in Bodybuilding* offers a sound, systematic, and *safe* approach to reaching your muscle potential through proper weight lifting.

There's been a fitness revolution in our country—and around the world—in recent decades. Countless millions of people jog, bike, swim, take aerobics classes, lift weights—you name it. We applaud all the different ways people choose to get in shape.

Bodybuilding, however, is unique and needs to be defined. Someone who goes to the gym occasionally and lifts a few weights for overall fitness is not a bodybuilder. Massive men with enormous bellies who compete in international weightlifting competitions are not bodybuilders.

Bodybuilding is all about developing and shaping your muscles—from the largest to the smallest, from your head to your toes. The goal is to sculpt your body little by little and eliminate any glaring deficiencies. Bodybuilders achieve impressive strength, but they probably wouldn't win a weightlifting contest against top-notch competitors. Bodybuilders are concerned with their overall look. They want to achieve the most muscular, proportional physique they can, not necessarily perform acts of great strength.

When some people think of bodybuilding, they recall competitions they've seen on TV, where contestants oil up their bodies to highlight their muscles, then flex and pose for judges who inspect their physique for the tiniest flaws. It's like a beauty contest—the best body wins.

Today, there are countless professional and amateur bodybuilding contests for men and women around the world. Some people get into bodybuilding with the intention of competing in contests and winning coveted titles. Others, however, have no interest in showing off their bodies onstage. They are drawn to the other rewards of bodybuilding—and there are many. For instance, bodybuilding can help you lose fat where it doesn't belong (stomach and thighs) while packing on muscles where they do belong (shoulders, chest, and arms). You can literally reshape your body.

Before long, your clothes fit better. You have more energy. You notice fewer aches and pains. You're more confident in your appearance. Your sex life may even improve!

As we age, we steadily lose muscle mass; starting at age 25, most people lose about a half-pound of muscle a year. Bodybuilding can reverse this process. It can actually help you gain muscle as you grow older. That's a pretty attractive proposition.

It's never too late to start strengthening and shaping your muscles. Many top bodybuilders began weight training in their early teens. That's perhaps the best time, because it allows you to develop a muscular foundation as your body matures. However, there are many famous bodybuilders who didn't start serious weight lifting until their late teens or early twenties.

In fact, you can start bodybuilding in your thirties or forties and make great gains. For that matter, some seniors—in their sixties, seventies, and beyond—pick up weights for the first time and discover renewed vigor and vitality. Weight training can boost your immune system, strengthen your bones, and improve the function of your heart and lungs. Lifting weights is as close to a fountain of youth as we've found.

One of the appeals of bodybuilding is that you can pursue it as far as you would like. You may begin training, start to look better in a t-shirt and shorts, and decide you don't want to develop bigger and bigger muscles. Your goal then becomes to maintain the gains you've made—and that's great.

Or you may experience an unparalleled rush from bodybuilding that drives you to pursue greater and greater results. You want larger muscles, better definition, more symmetry—more, more, more! Many of the world's best bodybuilders never imagined that they would become consumed with training and reach the pinnacle of their sport. Who knows—you could too!

This book is for anyone starting out in bodybuilding—no matter what his or her aspirations are. The truth is, everyone needs to learn the same training fundamentals, such as the proper lifting form, the right exercises to choose, and the optimum number of repetitions and sets. Without a good foundation, you're far more likely to suffer an injury or see mediocre results.

Then it's easy to become discouraged and abandon bodybuilding. One of our goals is to get you motivated and keep you motivated. That's done by encouraging you to follow an intelligent approach to training.

Good luck as you begin your bodybuilding mission. Keep in mind that *The Official Gold's Gym Guide to Getting Started in Bodybuilding* isn't intended to be read once and put on the shelf. Think of it as a reference book, a guide to lead you from beginning bodybuilding to the intermediate stage.

Don't be surprised if your progress seems slow, or even stagnant, at times. All top bodybuilders have low points in their training—when they question their methods, and even their desire. But the great ones press ahead and make adjustments in their workouts until gains resume and their enthusiasm returns.

*The Official Gold's Gym Guide to Getting Started in Bodybuilding* will give you the knowledge and confidence to analyze your training and make necessary changes from time to time. As top bodybuilders learn, training should become instinctive over time. You should be able to feel what works for you, as well as what doesn't. There's no one perfect regimen for everyone.

Listen to your body. Bodybuilding, done properly, should be as individual as you are.

# Getting Started

"I'm not exactly sure why I chose bodybuilding, except that I loved it. I loved it from the first moment my fingers closed around a barbell and I felt the challenge and exhilaration of hoisting the heavy steel plates above my head."

–Arnold Schwarzenegger, seven-time Mr. Olympia

Before we proceed, let's clear up a misconception about bodybuilding that has existed for years. The truth is:

**_Bodybuilding, done properly, does not make you stiff or muscle-bound_.**

In years past, coaches often discouraged athletes from lifting weights. They feared that large muscles would make the athletes bulky and slow instead of nimble and quick. Some players recognized the value of weight training, but often had to lift weights without their coach's knowledge.

Gradually, the benefits of muscle development have won coaches over in virtually every sport. Take baseball, for instance. Many of today's best hitters have physiques that rival those of many bodybuilders. Decades ago, by contrast, the best players often had thin, unimpressive builds. The word gradually spread in baseball, as well as in other sports, that proper weight lifting can improve—instead of inhibit—flexibility and speed. In addition, greater strength can increase stamina and durability.

Among non-athletes, however, there remain some people who think that bodybuilders, with all their mass, must be so muscle-bound that they can't even reach down to tie their shoes. Wrong! They ought to watch Flex Wheeler, one of today's top bodybuilders, as he does full splits onstage. That's right—full splits, with one leg extended straight in front and the other straight behind as he lowers himself to the floor.

We usually associate splits with tiny, pre-teen gymnasts blessed with incredible flexibility. Wheeler, by contrast, stands over six feet tall and weighs about 250 pounds in contest shape. His flexibility matches up with anybody's. So, to those who say "I don't want to start lifting weights because I might get too big," we say "Find another excuse."

Women, in particular, often fear that they'll become big and masculine-looking if they begin serious weight training. They don't want to look like a female version of Arnold Schwarzenegger. In fact, there is very little chance that a woman would ever resemble a male bodybuilder, even if she tried. Some women, it is true, have exceeded the bounds of femininity with their massive development, but these are the exception, not the rule, and many of them have relied on potentially dangerous drugs to boost their development. Women simply lack the genetic makeup to achieve the extreme muscularity of men.

Most women embrace bodybuilding in order to tone, shape, and firm their bodies—not to see how big they can make their muscles. Women often get just as much satisfaction from bodybuilding as men, but for different reasons. They find that it helps them manage their weight far better than yo-yo dieting does, and it helps them achieve a lean, graceful physique.

Women who lift weights are taken seriously today and are no longer viewed as oddities. Like men, they compete in prestigious bodybuilding contests around the world. Many famous actresses have trained with weights to prepare for demanding roles, thereby increasing the acceptance of female bodybuilding. As a result, women can now train in almost any gym without feeling uncomfortable. In fact, some of the world's top male bodybuilders now train side by side with their female counterparts. Equality has come to the weight room.

For both men and women, it's critical to get the proper start in bodybuilding. Many people fail to appreciate the demands and subtleties of weight lifting. They want to grab a barbell and start working out furiously in an attempt to reverse years of inactivity and get in shape—now!

There are right ways and wrong ways to begin bodybuilding. If you don't learn the proper weightlifting form, you can seriously injure your back, knees, or shoulders—virtually any part of your body. It takes time to become comfortable handling barbells and dumbbells (free weights). The sophisticated weight machines found in today's gyms can be easier to use, but they, like free weights, can be dangerous if used improperly.

Here's the best advice: start slowly. Use light weight at first until you master the correct lifting technique. Never bend from the waist and lift with your back. If you do, you risk back strain and perhaps chronic back trouble. Instead, bend at your knees and slowly lower yourself to the floor, keeping your back straight. Then grab the weight and gradually stand up. Now you're ready to begin your exercise.

Always lift in a smooth, controlled, rhythmic manner. Once you start, never make quick, jerky movements with a barbell or dumbbell. For instance, don't rock your body back and forth to try to lift heavy weight.

Don't try to impress others in the gym by showing how much weight you can lift. Form is far more important. If you try to lift too much weight, your form will suffer, and so will your results. Think of bodybuilding as a marathon, not a sprint. Look for gradual progress, not overnight miracles.

The key to successful bodybuilding is isolating specific muscles and working them to exhaustion. The muscles then recover and, over time, become stronger and larger. Different weightlifting exercises are designed to target different muscles. If you use your whole body during an exercise instead, you spread out the effort and fail to pinpoint one particular muscle. As a result, that muscle gets very little benefit.

It is far better to have several short workouts a week than one killer session that lasts hours and hours. A long workout might leave you so sore and exhausted that you would have to take time off to recover. If so, you could lose most of the gains you'd achieved.

Be patient. Be smart. To develop a systematic training regimen, follow the advice in *The Gold's Gym Guide to Getting Started in Bodybuilding.* If you learn good habits from the start, they'll always stay with you.

Here's another important point to consider as you begin bodybuilding: Genetics plays a key role in your ability to build a muscular physique. Anyone who trains properly over time can make impressive gains—but not everyone can become a champion bodybuilder.

It may seem unfair, but some people are born with a genetic makeup that lends itself to great muscularity. These people often train less than others, yet they achieve far greater results. You need to realistically assess your body before you begin serious training. You don't have to be naturally athletic in order to achieve bodybuilding success, but it helps.

Experts have identified three basic body types. Everyone fits more or less into one of these categories. Try to determine which body type best describes your frame.

- *Ectomorphs* naturally have a thin, wiry build with little body fat. They tend to have small muscles.

## BASIC EQUIPMENT

**Free weights:** barbells and dumbbells, the most basic weightlifting equipment. A barbell is a straight bar about 60 inches long. Dumbbells are much shorter, about 14 inches long. Weights are placed on the ends of both types of bars for resistance.

**Plates:** thin, circular weights that go on barbells and dumbbells. The lightest plates usually weigh 2.5 pounds, and plates increase in weight incrementally—5 pounds, 10 pounds, etc.—up to about 50 pounds each. You place a combination of different-sized plates on barbells and dumbbells to create the weight you want for an exercise.

**Collars:** metal devices of varying styles that are fastened on the ends of barbells and dumbbells to keep the plates in place.

**Machines:** the other type of equipment (besides barbells and dumbbells) that is used in weight lifting. Machines differ in size, shape, and complexity, using a combination of weights, pulleys, and cables. Typically, you sit on a bench, grab a handle, and push or pull a stack of weights. You select the amount of weight you want by inserting a metal pin in a specific position in the weight stack.

**Bench:** a basic piece of equipment used for many lifting exercises. *Flat benches,* for instance, are used in one of the most common chest exercises, Bench Press. Some exercises call for *incline benches,* in which the top of the bench is higher than the bottom. There are also *decline benches,* in which the bottom is higher than the top. Finally, there is a special bench called a *preacher bench* that is designed for Curls, a common biceps exercise.

**Gloves:** gloves, usually made of leather, that help you grip the bar better. They can also help reduce calluses, which are common among weight lifters. Often the palms of gloves are padded slightly to make lifting more comfortable. The fingers of a glove usually stop at the middle knuckle, allowing you to get your fingertips on the barbell, dumbbell, or machine for greater sensitivity and control.

**Weightlifting belt:** a wide, heavy belt, often made of leather or reinforced nylon. It helps stabilize your back and prevent injuries during heavy lifting. Some bodybuilders wear a belt while performing all their exercises. Others prefer to use a belt only when lifting maximum weight.

**Wraps:** cloth or elastic bands that you place around your elbows or knees during heavy lifting. Wraps support the joints and help you avoid injury.

**Log book:** a journal used to record workout regimen and progress. You write down which exercises you performed, the amount of weight used, the number of repetitions, etc. Logs can be very useful in planning workouts.

**Tape measure, scale, and camera:** tools used to document your weight and the size of your muscles before you begin bodybuilding so that you have a baseline by which to gauge your progress. Body weight can be deceiving because muscle weighs more than fat. It's possible to increase your weight at the same time that you're losing fat. Still, it's important to know your body weight as you begin. After weighing yourself, take measurements at your chest, shoulders, biceps, waist, thighs, and calves. Finally, get someone to take photos of you wearing shorts in several relaxed and flexed poses. As you make progress, you can compare yourself to the photos.

- *Endomorphs* are large and "doughy" by nature, with plenty of fat. They are stronger than ectomorphs, but their muscles aren't developed or defined.
- *Mesomorphs* are neither skinny nor fat. They have an attractive natural physique, and their muscles respond quickly to training. Most outstanding bodybuilders fit into this category.

Keep in mind that no one is entirely an ectomorph, an endomorph, or a mesomorph. Most of us have characteristics of all three, although one type is dominant. Why is this important? Your body type dictates the type of training you should do—and often predicts the results you'll achieve.

For instance, an ectomorph doesn't need to worry about losing fat to build a great physique, but he or she may struggle to develop and maintain large muscles. Don't get discouraged if you're an ectomorph. Some great bodybuilders have had this body type. Just understand that you may have to work harder to achieve your goals if you're thin by nature.

Endomorphs, on the other hand, may always fight a weight problem. However, their natural bulk can be an asset, too. If they train properly, they can awaken the muscles hidden beneath the fat and develop these muscles to great size. Many outstanding bodybuilders have been endomorphs.

Mesomorphs are the lucky ones. They typically don't have to fight the battle of the bulge or work out furiously to maintain their muscular development. They're capable of making rapid, impressive gains as soon as they begin serious training. Some top bodybuilders who are mesomorphs have won major titles within a few years of taking up the sport. However, don't get the idea that mesomorphs get a free ride. Just like ectomorphs and endomorphs, they have to work out intensely week after

week, month after month, year after year, to achieve greatness.

It's impossible to overemphasize the role of dedication and intensity in bodybuilding. These qualities are just as important—if not more so—than your body type. In any endeavor, people with enough "want to" can surpass people with more natural ability. The same is true for bodybuilding.

If you commit to a regular workout regimen—and train hard—you're assured of achieving respectable results. Intensity is critical. Some people love to go to the gym, but they don't really work out hard. They like to talk, look in the mirror, or stand by the water fountain. If they spend an hour in the gym, they think they've had a great workout. Not true.

Time in the gym doesn't necessarily equal results. Yes, some elite bodybuilders are known for spending four or five hours at a time working out, but that's generally not necessary. There are more great bodybuilders who spend only an hour or two at a time in the gym, but they know how to maximize every minute. They don't waste time with nonsense. Top bodybuilder Mike Matarazzo says, "When I train, it's like responding to a bell in boxing. Do your work and get out. Otherwise, you lose motivation and energy. I'm not a nice person in the gym."

One of the top female bodybuilders, Meryl Ertunc, agrees. "When I walk through the gym door, I start right in on my workout," she says. "I speak to nobody except my trainer. My sole objective is to focus on the workout and complete it effectively."

Because of differences in training intensity, it's hard to say how long you should work out. Thirty minutes? Forty-five minutes? An hour? As a general rule, if you start with a 45-minute workout three times a week, you'll make good progress. That will let you work all the major muscle groups and help you determine if you're an "easy gainer" or a "hard gainer." Some people, often because of their body type, see results far more quickly than others. They're "easy gainers."

By starting with shorter workouts, you'll also find out if you enjoy weight lifting. You won't become a great bodybuilder if you constantly have to force yourself to go to the gym. It may seem obvious, but you've got to like—or even love—weight training in order to sculpt a fantastic physique.

Bodybuilders who have left their mark in the sport couldn't stay away from the gym. For them, the problem was often *overtraining*—working out so often that they didn't give their bodies time to recover. We'll discuss overtraining later in the book, but it's a major problem for some people. You need to remember that proper rest and recovery are critical to making progress.

For now, don't worry about overtraining. Focus on learning to lift properly and becoming comfortable with weights. If overtraining ever becomes an issue, you can deal with it then.

## A BRIEF HISTORY OF BODYBUILDING

A century ago, the term "bodybuilder" didn't exist. Instead, men who showed off their muscles in public were called "strongmen."

Strongmen, popular in the late 1800s, specialized in performing acts of great strength—not developing picture-perfect bodies. Traveling carnivals often featured strongmen who performed a variety of stunts to the amazement of the carnival-goers. Their feats were impressive, but their physiques certainly were not. Many were bloated and overweight, with big guts and undefined muscles. In short, they would never be mistaken for today's bodybuilders.

A man named Eugen Sandow began to change the perception of strongmen. He, too, could perform acts of amazing strength, but he had a chiseled physique with little body fat—unlike other strongmen of the day. During the height of his popularity in the 1890s, Sandow traveled the country and posed for onlookers, often wearing only a fig

### TRAINING TERMS

**Burn:** the slightly painful, but also exhilarating, sensation that you get in a muscle at the end of a strenuous exercise.

**Muscle failure:** condition in which your muscles become so exhausted that you can't perform another repetition.

**Pump:** the dramatic muscle expansion after an intense exercise, before the muscles return to their normal size.

**Rep:** short for "repetitions." The number of reps is the number of times you complete an exercise movement.

**Ripped:** a term to describe extreme muscle definition. Bodybuilders try to become "ripped"—that is, develop muscles that stand out from others. Another term for ripped is "cut."

**Routine:** the sequence of exercises that make up a workout. Your routine, or regimen, will vary over time as you make progress and concentrate on different muscles.

**Set:** a group of repetitions. For instance, if you do eight reps of an exercise, that's one set. If you follow it up with another eight reps, that's two sets of eight reps.

**Spotter:** a person who stands beside you during an exercise to assist if necessary. A spotter can help you perform a final rep or two after your muscles become fatigued. Or a spotter can take a barbell from you if you've tried to lift too much.

**Training partner:** a person you work out with on a regular basis. Many bodybuilders have regular training partners. They find that partners help motivate them to achieve greater intensity during workouts. Partners can also serve as spotters.

**Vascularity:** the prominence of veins on a bodybuilder's well-developed physique. As a person becomes more "ripped," veins in the arms, chest, legs, and other areas begin to stand out.

leaf. People were intrigued by his unusual, impressive physique. When word spread that he trained with weights, sales of barbells took off for the first time.

Once Sandow achieved celebrity, other strongmen tried to build their bodies. In 1903, the first bodybuilding contest, called America's Most Perfectly Developed Man, was held at New York's Madison Square Garden. The winner took home the staggering sum (back then) of $1,000. The contest became an annual event, and the quality of contestants steadily improved.

In 1921, the winner was Angelo Siciliano, an Italian immigrant who afterwards changed his name to Charles Atlas. He was a marketing genius who developed a workout program called "dynamic tension"—aimed primarily at teenagers and young adults—and sold it in magazines and comic books.

In the now-famous Charles Atlas ads, a muscular bully kicks sand in the face of a skinny, pathetic-looking guy on the beach and then takes the guy's girlfriend. Angry, the "98-pound weakling" orders Atlas's dynamic tension program. He quickly builds rippling muscles and returns to the beach to beat up the bully and win back his girl. Sounds corny, but the pitch worked! Atlas made millions.

Ironically, Atlas built his own physique using traditional weightlifting methods, whereas the program sold to the "98-pound weakling" relied on isometrics. There was some merit to this approach, which involves flexing your muscles by pressing against stationary objects, but isometrics isn't nearly as effective as weight lifting. Still, Charles Atlas helped popularize bodybuilding.

The modern era of the sport began in the 1960s. Larry Scott, a handsome Californian, won the first two Mr. Olympia contests, held in 1965 and 1966. He wasn't particularly tall or massive by today's standards, but he developed the largest biceps anyone had seen in competition—close to 20 inches in circumference. Scott realized that nothing is more impressive on a bodybuilder than a huge set of "guns," or biceps. He developed a special incline bench to perform Curls, the standard biceps exercise. Today that piece of equipment is referred to as a "Scott bench" or "preacher bench."

Scott ushered in a wave of bodybuilders who grabbed the public's attention. One of the biggest names was Dave Draper, known as the Blond Bomber. Like Scott, he hailed from California and had movie star looks. By this time, muscle magazines had become popular, and Draper graced more covers than any other bodybuilder. He won the prestigious Mr. America title in 1965 and followed it up with Mr. Universe in 1966.

The next bodybuilding superstar was Sergio Oliva, a native of Cuba who defected to the United States during a bodybuilding competition. He was labeled The Myth for his awesome physique. He dominated bodybuilding in the mid- to late 1960s, winning the Mr. Olympia title from 1967 through 1969. Oliva had enormous shoulders, a chest that measured almost 60 inches (outstanding even today), and a waist that was only about 30 inches. To top it off, Olivia sported a mean, intimidating look that helped him "psych out" opponents in competition.

Oliva became the standard for bodybuilders—that is, until Arnold Schwarzenegger came on the scene in the late 1960s. Schwarzenegger, who emigrated from Austria, raised the bar. He had the most perfectly developed physique anyone had seen—and the charisma to match his body. More than any other bodybuilder, Arnold exposed the sport to the public and helped turn top bodybuilders into celebrities.

Arnold was featured in a highly acclaimed documentary about bodybuilding called *Pumping Iron,* released in 1976. The film followed Schwarzenegger and several competitors as they prepared for the previous year's Mr. Olympia contest.

Schwarzenegger helped inspire Lou Ferrigno, the next great bodybuilder. He was even bigger than Schwarzenegger, standing 6'5" tall and weighing 260 pounds. Ferrigno won all three major titles in the late 1970s—Mr. America, Mr. Olympia, and Mr. Universe—before following Arnold into show business.

After Ferrigno, top bodybuilders got even bigger and better. Today, their physiques are more defined and symmetrical than ever, thanks to ongoing advances in training techniques and diet. It's virtually impossible for the average observer to spot any weakness in today's top bodybuilders. Contests, as a result, are extremely competitive.

Where will the advances stop? Once, top bodybuilders weighed about 200 pounds. Today, they're pushing 300 pounds. You probably wouldn't want to get that big, even if you could—but you *can* benefit from the knowledge of world-class bodybuilders to craft the physique you've always wanted.

Evaluate your desire, set your goals, then go for it! Don't compare yourself to other bodybuilders. You are competing against yourself more than against anyone else.

## BEGINNING BODYBUILDING

When you begin weight lifting, you need to address two basic questions:

1. Where should I train?
2. Should I train alone or with a partner?

Today, good gyms are nearly everywhere. Finding a place to train is not nearly as difficult as it used to be. In shopping for a gym, however, location is critical. If you have to drive 45 minutes to get there, you probably won't go very often—and your progress will suffer. On the other hand, if the gym is just around the corner, you're much more likely to work out regularly.

Gyms, like people, have personalities. Some attract those who are interested in overall fitness. People who go to these gyms might want to take aerobics classes, do yoga, swim, or jog—but not necessarily lift weight. You can certainly pursue bodybuilding in a gym like this, as long as it has free weights and machines available. If you're the only bodybuilder in the gym, however, you may feel uncomfortable over time. As a result, your intensity—and the frequency of your workouts—may wane.

If you really intend to be a serious bodybuilder, you're probably better off joining a gym that's geared toward "ironheads," fellow hard-core lifters. These folks normally don't care about fancy dressing areas, saunas, or aerobics classes. They're only interested in rows and rows of barbells and machines. Does that describe you? If you're an ironhead, you'll thrive in an environment like this. You'll be more likely to train with intensity because others are training hard, too.

These days, some people choose to train at home instead of joining a gym. It's now possible to buy first-class, gym-quality workout equipment for your home, because it has come down enough in both price and size that it's practical to keep in a spare bedroom. However, before you shell out thousands of dollars for equipment, buy an inexpensive barbell set, which can cost $50 to $100. A basic barbell set will allow you to learn the proper lifting form, get used to handling weights, and find out if you really enjoy weight training—and if you like working out at home. If so, you can steadily add to and upgrade your equipment.

## BODYBUILDING BIO:
## Arnold Schwarzenegger

Schwarzenegger is one of the few bodybuilding celebrities identified by first name alone.

Mention "Arnold" and the subject of bodybuilding, and there's no doubt who you mean. He's the most dominant and influential bodybuilder in history. Even today—20 years after he retired from competition—Arnold towers over current bodybuilding champions in terms of public awareness.

His rise to stardom epitomizes the American dream. Born and raised in a small Austrian village, he was exposed to weight lifting for the first time when he was 14 years old. He was mesmerized.

"I still remember the first visit to the bodybuilding gym," he writes in his 1977 autobiography, *Arnold: The Education of a Bodybuilder.* "Those guys were huge and brutal. I found myself walking around them, staring at muscles I couldn't even name, muscles I'd never even seen before.

"The weightlifters shone with sweat; they were powerful looking, Herculean. And there it was before me—my life, the answer I'd been seeking."

Even at a young age, he knew that he wanted to be a bodybuilder—the best ever. He didn't speak English at the time, yet he imagined coming to America, achieving bodybuilding fame, and using it to achieve success in other fields. He didn't let the skepticism of other people discourage him.

"With my desire and my drive, I definitely wasn't normal," Arnold wrote. "Normal people can be happy with a regular life. I felt there was more to life than just plodding through an average existence.

"I'd always been impressed with stories of greatness and power. Caesar, Charlemagne, Napoleon were names I knew and remembered. . . . I saw bodybuilding as the vehicle that would take me to the top, and I put all my energy into it."

Before he could dedicate himself solely to bodybuilding, however, Arnold had to serve a year in the Austrian army. From age 18 to 19 he was stationed at an army camp, yet he still found time to train intensely.

He went AWOL to compete in the 1965 Junior Mr. Europe competition in Stuttgart, Germany. "The contest meant so much to me that I didn't care what consequences I'd have to suffer," Arnold wrote. "I crawled over the wall, taking only the clothes I was wearing. I had barely enough money to buy a third-class train ticket."

He borrowed an outfit to compete in, and he won the title. When he returned to the army camp, the officers weren't impressed with his trophy. They confined him in a military jail for a week with little food.

Slowly, however, others at the camp recognized Arnold's extraordinary talent and desire. Superiors encouraged him to train and relieved him of some normal responsibilities. They held him up as an example for other young men to follow. "I became a hero, even though I had defied their rules to get what I wanted," he wrote.

The next year, with his confidence buoyed, Arnold entered the 1966 Mr. Universe contest. The competition was much fiercer. "I had assumed that after almost five years of training, I knew all there was to know about bodybuilding," he wrote. "As it turned out, I knew next to nothing."

He said he took one look at the eventual winner, Chet Yorton, and realized how far he had to go. "He had all the qualities it took to be Mr. Universe—the muscularity, the separation, the definition, the skin color, the glow of confidence," Arnold wrote. "He was finished, like a piece of sculpture ready to be put on display."

Arnold didn't despair. He began training harder than ever and won the next Mr. Universe contest in 1967. His period of dominance had begun. Starting in 1970, Arnold won bodybuilding's top prize—Mr. Olympia—for six straight years.

Then he turned to a new challenge—acting. His first film, *Conan the Barbarian* in 1980, was a moderate success, but he used it as a springboard to eventually become a top box-office draw.

Over the years, Arnold has never strayed far from bodybuilding. After completing *Conan the Barbarian,* he returned from a five-year retirement from the sport to win his seventh and final Mr. Olympia title in 1980. A few competitors groused that Arnold won on his name alone, that his physique was no longer the best. No matter. Arnold took home the title—and further cemented his role as bodybuilding's ruler.

In 1994, he began sponsoring a bodybuilding competition that has become an annual event. The Arnold Classic Weekend features contests for men and women and always draws a large field. Arnold says he's encouraged by today's bodybuilders and optimistic about the sport's future.

"Bodybuilding is so specialized and so difficult that only a small percentage of people will ever want to do what it takes to become an international champion," he wrote in *The New Encyclopedia of Bodybuilding,* published in 1998. "But athletes who once would have been drawn to other sports are now beginning to consider a career in bodybuilding.

"This is one of the things that will ensure that the sport will continue to grow, that the level of competition will remain high, and that the public's interest will continue to increase."

Virtually all serious bodybuilders, however, eventually train at a gym. The reasons are obvious. Good gyms have a far more extensive assortment of weights and machines than you could probably afford to buy for your home. At a gym, you also have plenty of people to "spot" you—that is, lend a hand if you've grabbed too much weight.

This leads to the question of a training partner. Do you need one? There's no answer that's right for everyone. Perhaps you thrive on the rapport that develops between regular training buddies. If you know someone is waiting for you at the gym, you may be more likely to show up; you may also be likely to train harder. In addition, some exercises are difficult (and may even be dangerous) to perform alone.

Still, there are valid reasons *not* to have a training partner. Perhaps you're self-motivated and don't need anyone else to fuel your intensity. Working with a partner might slow your workouts and impede your progress. Bodybuilding, after all, is fundamentally an individual sport.

Give it some thought. You probably already have an idea whether you'd benefit from a training partner—or not.

Another critical element in bodybuilding is diet. We'll devote an entire chapter to nutrition and diet later, but keep in mind that what you eat has a huge effect on your muscle development.

If you're undisciplined in your eating—and if you have no desire to change—you severely limit your chances for success. You don't have to become a food fanatic or take lots of expensive, exotic supplements, but you do need to pay attention to your food intake. Without an awareness of what you eat, as well as when and how much you eat, you won't be able to make the dietary adjustments necessary for peak muscle development.

Many bodybuilders swear by dietary supplements, but the best supplements in the world can't take the place of intense, regular training. There's no such thing as a magic elixir or a "workout in a jar," so beware of products that promise unbelievable results. Like the saying goes, "If it sounds too good to be true, it probably is."

Besides being ineffective, supplements may contain unproven and even dangerous ingredients. For advanced bodybuilders with a thorough knowledge of nutrition, supplements can be useful and provide an extra edge in competition. Just don't begin bodybuilding with the idea that a pill or a powder can take the place of dedication and sweat. There are no shortcuts.

Finally, before you start serious weight training, be sure to get a thorough physical exam. Even young people can have potentially serious health problems that are undiagnosed. A checkup is usually quick, easy, and inexpensive. When it's over, you'll have the peace of mind to let you train your hardest.

# 2

## Your First Routines

"The name of the game in bodybuilding is intensity. There's absolutely
no question that increased training intensity develops more massive muscles
and better muscle quality."

—Tom Platz, former Mr. Universe

All top bodybuilders learn to tailor their workouts to what's effective for them and what helps them achieve their goals.

Because no two people are alike, exercises that work great for one bodybuilder may produce poor results for another. As you gain experience, you'll learn which exercises are best for you and how to structure your workouts.

Still, when starting out, everyone should become familiar with some well-established, basic weightlifting exercises. These cover all the major muscle groups: shoulder, chest, arm, leg, and abdomen. Once you become comfortable with these—and notice how your muscles respond—you'll be in a position to customize your routines.

These 19 basic exercises provide the foundation on which you can develop your bodybuilder's physique. Tried-and-true exercises such as Bench Press, Curls, and Squats are so effective that even champion bodybuilders never abandon them entirely. Top competitors constantly tinker with their regimen, trying different exercises that

they hope will take them to the next level, but they never stray far from the core exercises that they mastered as beginners.

Take a lesson from the pros. Learn these basic exercises by heart. And keep this in mind: Look for steady, consistent progress, not overnight miracles. Many budding bodybuilders, unfortunately, have unrealistic expectations and underestimate the time it will take to reshape their physiques. Many people, sadly, become discouraged and give up bodybuilding before they ever discover their potential. The prize in bodybuilding—as in most endeavors—usually goes to the turtle, not the hare.

With that said, let's recap some of the appeals of bodybuilding to energize you as you begin.

While none of us can control our genes—nature has predetermined our height and body shape to a large extent—each of us *can* improve the body we were born with, and there's no better way to do this than weight lifting.

Most bodybuilders choose the sport because they feel they are too skinny or too fat, or they may simply feel that they have a mediocre build. Weight lifting lets you sculpt and reshape your body. By choosing the right exercises and performing them properly, you can add muscle here, lose fat there, and tone up from head to toe.

## STRETCHING AND WARMING UP

Top athletes in all sports know the importance of stretching and preparing their bodies for a strenuous workout. If you don't stretch, you're far more likely to strain a muscle, ligament, or tendon. Even a mild injury can keep you out of the gym for several days or weeks, significantly slowing down your progress.

Weight training, even when done properly, places tremendous stress on your body. While the stress of resistance to weight is what leads to muscle growth, lifting heavy weights can damage your body if you haven't prepared it properly.

That's where warming up and stretching come in. They are actually two different steps, although they're often lumped together.

Warming up involves motion. The best example is light aerobic activity, such as riding a stationary bike or walking on a treadmill. The purpose is to elevate your heart rate, boost your

### BODYBUILDER BIO: Lee Haney

Lee Haney turned disappointment in one sport into a record-setting career in another.

Lee began bodybuilding after he broke a leg playing high school football in South Carolina. Like many teens, Lee had aspirations of playing professional football—and he had the talent to make that dream come true. But while rehabilitating his injured leg in the weight room he discovered that he liked lifting weights more than playing football.

"They sent me into the weight room to rehabilitate my atrophied leg muscles, and I never came out again," Lee said. "Once I had experienced the thrill of being able to add muscle mass to my frame, I was an ex-footballer and a lifetime bodybuilder."

Lee found that his body quickly responded to weight training, and he liked his new muscle mass. He could quickly envision success as a bodybuilder.

It turns out that he was right.

"Large Lee," as he became known, won eight straight Mr. Olympia titles from 1984 to 1991. That's bodybuilding's top prize, akin to the Super Bowl in pro football. Lee even bettered the previous record of seven Mr. Olympia wins by the incomparable Arnold Schwarzenegger. Many people had thought Arnold's record would never be broken.

Lee started serious weight training when he was 16 years old and soon began winning youth bodybuilding contests. A photo of him at age 17 shows what an extraordinary physique he had already developed.

Lee began accumulating national bodybuilding titles in 1979 when he won Teen Mr. America. He followed it up with victories in the 1982 Junior Nationals bodybuilding contest and the World Amateur Championships later that year.

In 1983, he entered his first Mr. Olympia contest and shocked people by finishing third—much higher than most competitors do on their first attempt. Still, he wasn't content. The judges' comments noted that his arms and calves were too small, and he set out to correct those flaws in his physique.

The next year, he won the Mr. Olympia title—blowing away the field. Lee's dominance in bodybuilding had begun.

Throughout his career, he was known for his intense workouts and the incredible size he achieved. He was especially known for his massive back, which seemed to dwarf the backs of other competitors. Standing just under 6 feet tall, he carried 250 pounds of rippling muscle in contest shape.

Today Lee is retired and lives outside Atlanta, Georgia. He owns a 40-acre ranch that he calls "Haney's Harvest House," and he works with inner-city youth. He's one of the leading promoters of bodybuilding: He saw what it did for him, and he knows what it can do for others, in terms of both physique and self-esteem.

"Every bodybuilder wants to develop huge, powerful muscles," says Lee, now 43. "In fact, that's usually the main reason why most of us started working out with weights in the first place—to build up a skinny frame so we could look huge and powerful. No matter how massive a bodybuilder gets, he still wants to add a little more muscle to certain parts of his physique."

breathing, and get your blood pumping harder. You're literally "warming up" your body for a full workout.

Stretching, on the other hand, is static—that is, you stand or sit in place as you slowly extend your muscles to make them more limber. The more you can stretch your muscles, the larger they can become.

Most experts recommend that you warm up before you stretch. Why? If you stretch when your body is cold, you're far more likely to pull a muscle. A good warm-up should take about 10 minutes—long enough to work up a light sweat but not so long that you become fatigued and have less energy for your upcoming weight training.

Once you've warmed up, it's time to stretch. Stretching is intended to increase your flexibility and reduce injuries during lifting.

It's tempting to bypass stretching if you're in a hurry and want to start lifting immediately, but that's a mistake. "I stretch out a lot," says top bodybuilder Mike Matarazzo. "You've got to stay loose. Whatever muscles you're working, find a way to stretch them." Particularly as we get older, we need to properly prepare our bodies for demanding workouts to avoid injury and to get the most benefit. Don't shortchange yourself.

Stretching has other benefits besides cutting down on injuries. It helps to relieve tension and focuses your mind on your approaching workout. Stretching also lengthens your muscles and gives you a leaner, more toned appearance—a huge asset for competition. "Many people don't realize the value of stretching to strengthen and elongate the muscle and help it grow," said Lee Labrada, two-time Mr. Olympia runner-up.

Stretching, however, must be done properly. It should always be gradual and gentle, with no bouncing or jerking movements. It may take up to 30 seconds to reach the fully stretched position, and if you rush it you won't get the full benefit.

Stretching is a good pre-workout activity, but many bodybuilders also stretch *during* and *after* workouts. Muscles can become tense and tight during intense lifting, and stretching during a workout can help make them limber and ready to lift some more.

After a workout, stretching is an excellent way to cool down. For one thing, it's much easier on your body to bring your heart and breathing rates down gradually than to stop exercising suddenly. In addition, stretching after a workout helps prevent muscle soreness and promotes faster muscle recovery. It's after a workout, as your muscles recover, that most muscle growth actually occurs.

## Names of Muscles
### Upper Body
- Pectorals ("pecs"—chest muscles)
- Deltoids ("delts"—rounded muscles at the top of the shoulders)
- Latissimus dorsi muscles ("lats"—muscles extending from under the armpits across the back to the spine)
- Trapezius muscles ("traps"—muscles extending from the neck to the middle of the back)
- Spinal erectors (horizontal muscles extending down the back to just above the waist)
- Obliques (muscles on the side of the torso, next to the abdominals)
- Intercostals (diagonal muscles across the ribs, just above the abdominals)
- Serratus muscles (diagonal muscles slightly above the intercostals, near the pectorals)
- Abdominals ("abs"—vertical muscles extending the length of the abdomen)

### Arms
- Biceps
- Triceps

- Forearm flexors (muscles of the inside of the forearm)
- Forearm extensors (muscles of the outside of the forearm)

### Legs
- Quadriceps ("quads"—muscles at the front of the thigh)
- Hamstrings (muscles that extend from the back of the thigh to the lower leg)
- Gastrocnemius muscles (upper calf muscles)
- Soleus muscles (lower calf muscles)

### Buttocks
- Gluteus maximus muscles ("glutes"—muscles of the buttocks)

## STRETCHING EXERCISES

The following basic stretching exercises cover all the major muscle groups.

### Standing Torso Bend
*Area worked:* Obliques

*Instructions:* Stand with your feet slightly more than shoulder-width apart and your arms at your sides. Raise your right arm overhead, bent at the elbow. Keep your arm there and lean your torso to the left as far as possible while keeping your feet stable. To lean farther, slide your left arm down the outside of your left leg. Hold this position for about 15 seconds, then return to start-

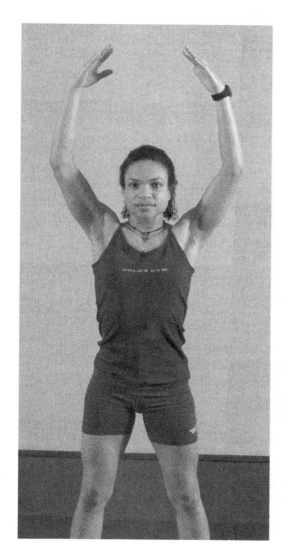
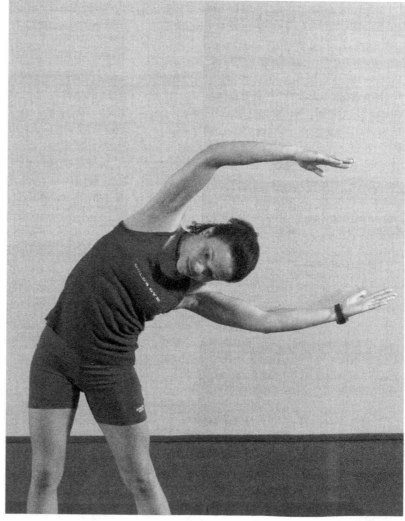

**Standing Torso Bend**

ing position. Repeat with your left arm overhead and lean to the right. You may also do the exercise with both arms raised overhead at the same time.

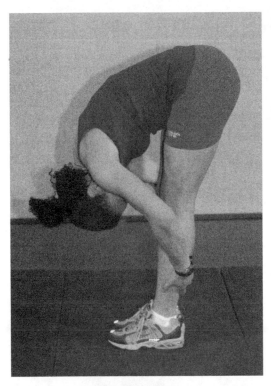

**Forward Bend**

### Forward Bend

*Areas worked:* Lower back, hamstrings

*Instructions:* Stand upright, with your feet together. Bend forward gradually and grab the backs of your calves. Slowly try to reach down farther. See if you can touch the backs of your ankles, but don't strain. Lower your head toward your shins to let you reach farther down. When you're at the lowest point you can comfortably maintain, hold the position for 30 seconds.

### Seated Torso Bend

*Areas worked:* Obliques, lower back, spine

*Instructions:* Sit on the floor with your legs extended in front of you. Bend your right leg up so your knee is chest high, keeping your left leg on the floor. Twist your torso to the right as far as possible while keeping your buttocks on the floor. Extend your right arm behind you for support. To help you twist, place your left elbow on the outside of your right knee. When you've twisted as far as possible, hold

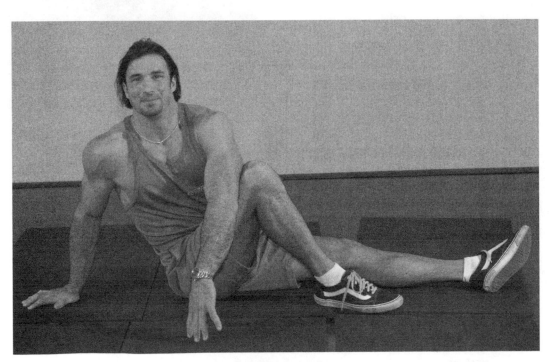

**Seated Torso Bend**

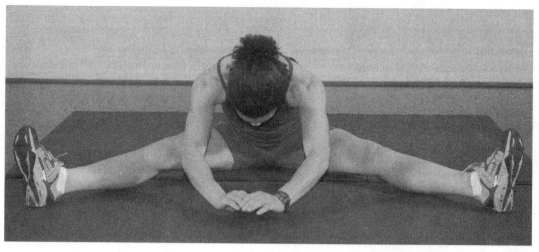

**V-Stretch**

the position for 30 seconds. Then repeat with your left leg bent at the knee, and twist to the left.

### V-Stretch

*Areas worked:* Hamstrings, lower back

*Instructions:* Sit on the floor with your knees locked and legs extended in a wide V. Bend forward and extend your arms in front of you as far as possible. With your fingers touching the floor, hold the position for 10 seconds. Then gradually turn to your right and grab your right ankle. Hold for 10 seconds. Return to the starting position. Then turn and grab your left ankle, holding for 10 seconds.

### Lunges

*Areas worked:* Inner thighs, glutes
*Instructions:* Crouch on the floor with your left leg extended behind you and your right leg bent so the thigh is parallel to the floor. Lean forward until your torso touches your right thigh. Place the fingers of both hands on the floor, directly below your shoulders. Hold your head up and look straight ahead. Hold for 15 seconds, stretching your torso forward and down. Stand, returning to the starting position. Repeat with your right leg behind you and your left leg bent.

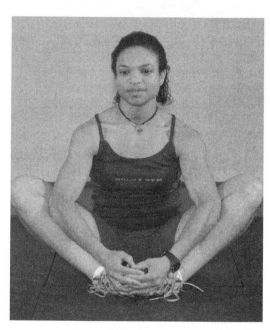

**Groin Stretch**

### Groin Stretch

*Areas worked:* Groin muscles, inner thighs

*Instructions:* Sit on the floor with your knees bent and turned outward. Pull your feet as close to your buttocks as possible. Grab the outer front edges of your feet, and rest your elbows on your thighs. *Slowly* press down on your legs, lowering them closer to the floor. (Don't press too far. Your knees should stop about a foot from the floor.) At the lowest point, hold for 15 seconds.

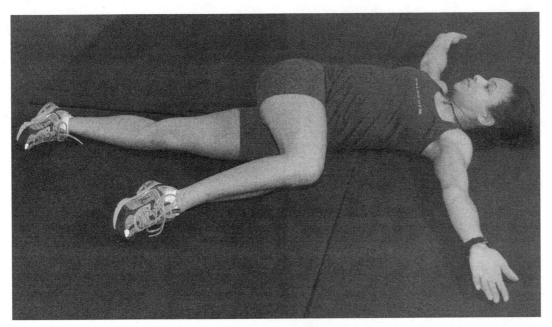

**Leg Crossover**

### Leg Crossover

*Areas worked:* Lower back, hips, thighs

*Instructions:* Lie on your back with your legs together and straight. Extend your arms to the side at a 90-degree angle to your torso. While keeping your arms stationary, lift your right leg straight up, then cross it over your left leg. Touch your right toes to the floor, even with your knee. (It is important to keep your arms and left leg stationary for maximum benefit.) Hold for 15 seconds. Repeat, lifting your left leg and crossing it over your right leg.

### Back Roll

*Area worked:* Mid-back

*Instructions:* Lie on your back with your knees pulled against your chest. Grab the upper part of your shins and gradually press your legs toward your chest. Hold for 15 seconds. Then, *gradually* rock backward until your weight rests on your shoulder blades. Be sure to keep your balance. Keep your hands on your legs. (*Caution:* If this is uncomfortable, don't do it. Roll forward until your weight is on your back again.) Hold for 15 seconds.

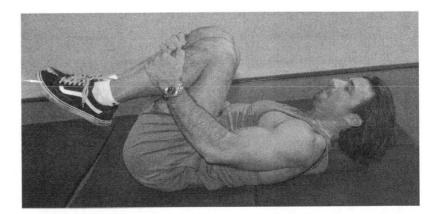

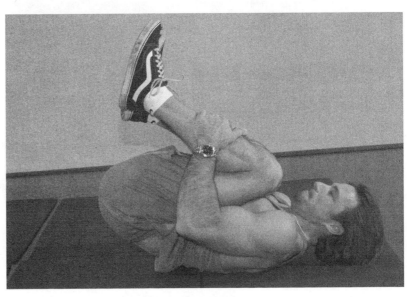

**Back Roll**

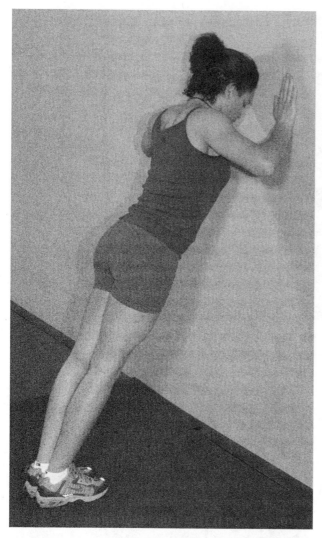

**Calf Stretch**

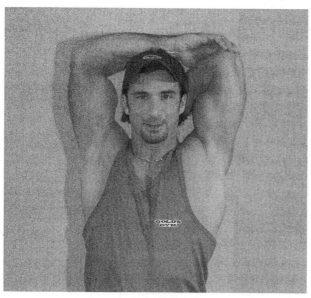

**Triceps Stretch**

### Calf Stretch

*Area worked:* Calves

*Instructions:* Stand about an arm's length from a wall. Lean forward and place both palms on the wall. Keep your legs straight and together. Slowly lean your head forward until it touches the wall. Keep your feet flat on the floor and feel your calf muscles stretch. Hold for 15 seconds. Then rise up on your toes to stretch farther. Hold for another 15 seconds.

### Triceps Stretch

*Area worked:* Triceps

*Instructions:* Stand with your feet about shoulder-width apart. Raise your left arm and bend it at the elbow. Place your left hand behind your head on your right shoulder blade. Your left forearm should be against your head. With your right hand, gently press down on your left elbow. Your left hand should move down slightly. At the lowest point you can comfortably maintain, hold for 15 seconds. Repeat with your right arm behind your head, pressing down with your left hand.

### Crunches

*Area worked:* Abs

*Instructions:* Lie on your back on the floor in front of a flat bench. Bend your knees and place the backs of your calves on top of the bench. Clasp your hands behind your head. Exhale and raise your head and shoulders toward your knees, keeping your back on the floor. Inhale and lower yourself to the floor. Repeat. (This is a very short movement. It's not a full sit-up, in which you touch your elbows to your knees. It's critical to do it slowly and deliberately in order to get the full effect.)

### Neck Roll

*Area worked:* Neck

*Instructions:* Stand with your feet about shoulder-width apart. Place your

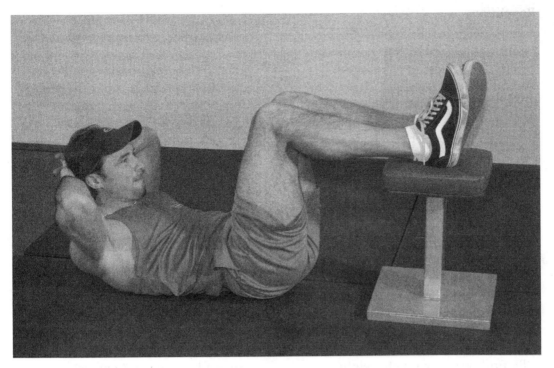

**Crunches**

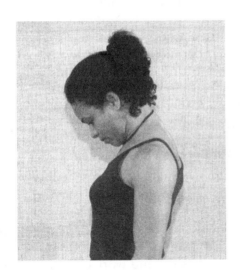
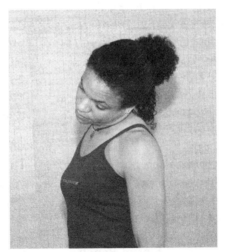
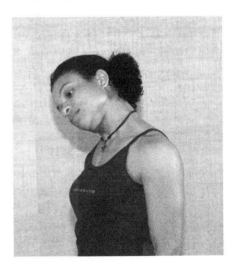

**Neck Roll**

palms on either side of your waist or let your arms hang straight down. Bend your head forward until your chin almost touches your chest. Hold for 15 seconds. Then slowly rotate your head to the right, making a complete circle around your body. Do this 3 times, slowly. Then reverse and rotate your head to the left, making a circle 3 times.

## LIFTING BASICS

Before we present the basic weightlifting exercises, we need to address several issues about training. These include the correct number of repetitions and sets to do, correct breathing, the length and frequency of your workouts, warm-up sets, and what to do about soreness.

## Repetitions

Select a weight that allows you to comfortably do 8 to 10 repetitions, or reps, regardless of the exercise. As you become stronger, work up to 12 to 15 reps. At that point, it's time to add more weight (5 or 10 pounds) and drop the number of reps back to 8 to 10. Then work up to 12 to 15 reps at the heavier weight. That's the cycle to follow as you progress in weight training—increase reps, then add weight.

As a general rule, work out with about 75% of the weight that you could lift one time. For instance, if you can bench press 100 pounds once, you should work out with about 75 pounds and do 8 to 10 reps.

However, there's no need to repeatedly find out how much weight you can lift one time. After all, you're not training to be a power lifter, where lifting maximum weight is the goal. You're interested in being a bodybuilder, where muscle development is the objective. This is achieved by doing multiple reps in a smooth, rhythmic manner with a weight you can handle.

## Sets

Some people confuse sets and repetitions. The number of reps is the number of times you lift a weight. The number of sets is the number of times you complete an exercise. For instance, if you do 10 reps of Bench Press, that's one set. If you follow up with 10 more reps, that's two sets—and so on.

As a beginner, you should start with two sets per exercise, although it would be fine to do just one set until you become comfortable with lifting. Experienced bodybuilders may do 10 or more sets of an exercise, but some experts believe that doing so many sets becomes counterproductive. Once you gain experience, you can do more sets. For now, limit yourself to two, resting about one minute between sets.

The number of sets you do is less important than your intensity while lifting. "More [sets] aren't better," says Paul DeMayo, a top bodybuilder. "It's what you do in the amount of time. I don't hang around. People are amazed that I make progress because they're convinced you have to be in there four, five, six hours a day."

## Breathing

Many beginning weight lifters don't breathe properly. There's a natural tendency to hold your breath as you perform an exercise, but that can be dangerous. You can become so weak and dizzy that you pass out.

Instead, inhale and exhale in a smooth, steady manner. Inhale during the easier part of an exercise (when you're lowering the weight) and exhale during the harder part (lifting). Your breathing should work in harmony with your lifting. Proper breathing will quickly become second nature, and then you won't have to think about it anymore.

## Workout Duration and Frequency

There are two main ways to schedule your workouts. You can train all your muscles three times a week—such as on Monday, Wednesday, and Friday—or you can train only some of your muscles at a time and work out six days a week. The choice is yours. Just be sure not to train seven days a week. Your muscles need at least one day to recover and grow.

Some people like the sensation of working all their muscles at once, then taking a day off before doing a full-body workout again. Others, however, like to concentrate on certain muscles—such as the shoulders, chest, and back—one day, then concentrate on other muscles the next day. They think it helps their intensity to work only certain muscles at a time.

If you choose to train six days a week, be sure to keep your workouts short. If you lift for too long, you can become so tired that your form suffers.

As a beginner, you can do an excellent workout in 45 minutes if you're focused. That allows enough time to do exercises that cover all the major muscle groups. Once you become more experienced, you can extend your workouts by increasing the number of sets and exercises.

The length of your workouts may vary to some degree, depending on whether you use free weights— barbells and dumbbells—or machines. It usually takes longer to lift with free weights because you have to add and remove weight plates between exercises. With machines, you simply place a pin in the weight stack and start lifting.

Many elite bodybuilders train almost exclusively with free weights because they believe that barbells and dumbbells allow them more variety in their workouts. For instance, machines generally limit the lifting motion; that is, the weights travel only along a certain path. With free weights, you can vary

## BODYBUILDER BIO: Dorian Yates

After Lee Haney retired with a record eight straight Mr. Olympia titles, Dorian Yates of England started a streak of his own. Beginning in 1992, Yates won the Mr. Olympia title six consecutive times.

Many believe that he displayed an even better physique than Haney. Lee weighed about 250 pounds, but Yates topped the scales at 265 to 270—with a body fat percentage in the single digits.

Yates' granite-like build is even more impressive considering that he didn't begin bodybuilding until he was almost 20 years old. By his own admission, he was a troublemaker during his childhood in a small village outside Birmingham, England. He often hung around in clubs with groups of skinheads, he says.

But a short stint in jail for disorderly conduct turned Yates' life around. He began weight lifting and, like many bodybuilding champs, became instantly addicted to it.

"When I first began bodybuilding, I immediately knew that it was for me," says Yates, now 41. "I read as much as I could about training, nutrition, and anything else that would help me succeed as a bodybuilder. Once I found the things that interested me, I'd give them a try in the gym."

Early on, Yates showed the intelligence that it takes to excel in bodybuilding. He paid attention to which exercises worked best for him, and he set his routines accordingly. "Through a lot of trial and error, I found the training system and diet that worked for me," Yates says.

Some people are surprised to learn that Yates, despite his enormous size, never spent hours and hours at a time in the gym. He found that fewer sets worked better for him. For example, he limited himself to 6 to 8 sets per body part. Granted, that's a lot for a beginner—more than you should try. But it's far fewer sets than some top bodybuilders do.

"The most common mistake made by eager bodybuilders is overtraining," Yates says. "I regularly see beginners doing 15 to 20 sets of chest work and wondering why their pecs aren't growing. It's only by avoiding the pitfalls of constant overtraining that I have been able to make good gains in the chest area."

Yates says intensity is far more important than the number of sets you do. "Most bodybuilders are overtrained in sets and undertrained in intensity," he says. "My advice is to cut the number of exercises and sets you are doing by 50% and double your intensity. Then watch what happens."

He says beginners shouldn't try to lift too much weight, but should use a weight that they can handle and still maintain good lifting form. "Training is not just about heavy weights," Yates says. "It's also about really clean form, full mental involvement and taking the muscles to the point of failure."

He says he became a bodybuilder because he enjoyed it, not to impress others with his massive physique. "The general public perception of bodybuilding is that it is an egotistical, narcissistic sport," Yates says. "Maybe it is, but I never approached it from that point of view. I was never into trying to get people's adulation.

"I never walked around in a tank top and never wanted people to notice me or adore me. I didn't ever build my body for that reason. I did it for myself."

the lifting motion almost infinitely to achieve your goals.

Machines, however, do have advantages. You can perform some very effective exercises on machines that are difficult to do with free weights. In addition, using machines is often safer because you don't have to support the full weight as you do with a barbell.

Regardless of how you plan your workout, or whether you use free weights or machines, it's important to determine what time of day is best for you to train and then to establish a regular routine.

Some people have more energy in the morning and like to work out then. Others are more alert later in the day or at night. It's not the time of day that matters. *Intensity* matters. If you can work out harder at 7 A.M., that's the time to do it. If you can train harder at 7 P.M., that's the time to do it. Either way, establish a routine. Don't work out at 6 A.M. one day, at 10 P.M. the next, and at noon the following day. Your body needs a regular schedule.

As you do your workouts, remember that progress in bodybuilding rarely occurs on a straight-line continuum. Instead, you'll probably make gains in spurts. You may go weeks or even months without any noticeable improvement. If you keep training, however, the gains will return.

Just be consistent and don't make excuses to skip workouts. "Unless you are so ill that you must remain in bed, you should never miss a scheduled workout," says Boyer Coe, a former Mr. Universe. "One missed workout can set your progress back by as much as a week, because you actually experience negative results from missing a training session."

### Warm-Up Sets

Earlier we discussed warming up before a workout. Ideally, you should do 5 to 10 minutes of light aerobic activity, such as riding a stationary bike or using a stair machine. This prepares your body for lifting.

There's another kind of warm-up that's just as critical: warm-up sets. This involves doing sets with light weight before you perform the same exercise with your regular training weight. For warm-up sets, use about half the weight and do about twice as many reps. If you normally do 8 reps of Bench Press with 150 pounds, warm up by doing 15 reps with 75 pounds.

With the lighter weight and higher reps, you can concentrate on proper lifting form and prepare your muscles for the heavier weight.

As you become more advanced, warm-up sets are even more critical. Some competitive bodybuilders who use extremely heavy weight do several warm-up sets for each exercise. This helps them avoid injury.

### Soreness vs. Pain

Muscle soreness is a natural part of bodybuilding. In fact, moderate soreness is an indicator that you're doing exercises correctly and making progress. There's an exhilarating, satisfying feel to an intense workout that leaves your muscles pumped and sore. The soreness will go away in a day or two and won't interfere with your next workout.

However, *pain* isn't a good sign, so it's important to learn to tell the difference between soreness and pain. For example, if your back hurts so much that you can barely stand up, that pain is the result of improper lifting. Pain is a warning sign that you might be causing an injury that could sideline you for weeks. If you feel a sharp, sudden pain during lifting, stop immediately. By doing so, you're not being a wimp—you're being *smart*. If the pain persists, seek medical attention.

"No pain, no gain" is a popular term in sports. We might amend it for bodybuilding to "No soreness, no gain."

## BASIC EXERCISES

### Upper Body

#### Bench Press

*Primary muscles used:* Chest

*Technique:* Lie on a flat bench that has uprights to hold a barbell. Place your feet on the floor at the end of the bench. Grab the bar above your head with an overhand grip (palms down, thumbs in) and with your hands placed slightly more than shoulder-width apart. Lift the bar straight up off the

**WORDS TO TRAIN BY**

"To make a muscle grow, you must force it to go beyond its capabilities. The most potent way to apply that force is to train to failure. Training to failure means . . . the muscles are forced to grow stronger and bigger."

—Nasser El Sonbaty, an international bodybuilding star

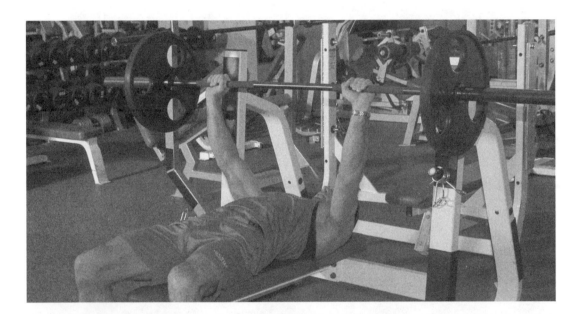

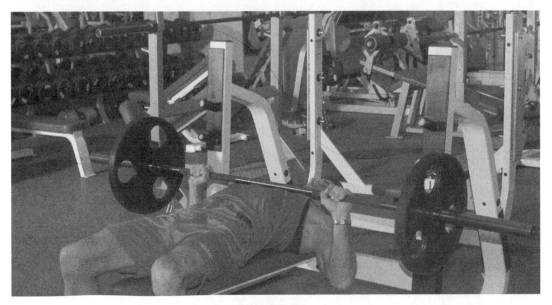

**Bench Press**

supports, locking your elbows. Exhale as you lift. Then inhale and slowly lower the bar until it touches the highest point of your chest. Let the bar rest there for a second, then exhale and push the bar straight up, locking your elbows again. Repeat.

### Dumbbell Flye

*Primary muscles used:* Chest

*Technique:* Lie on a flat bench with no supports for a barbell. Grab a dumb-bell in each hand, with your arms extended and even with the top of the bench. Bend your elbows slightly. Then raise the dumbbells in front of you, in line with your chest, until they touch. Make sure you have a secure grip, then exhale and lower the dumb-bells to your sides (along the same path) until they are even with the top of the bench. Hold for a second, then exhale and lift the dumbbells again until they touch. Repeat.

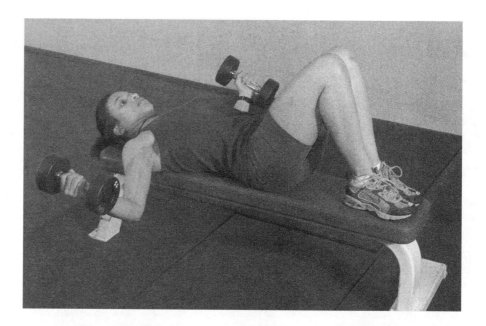

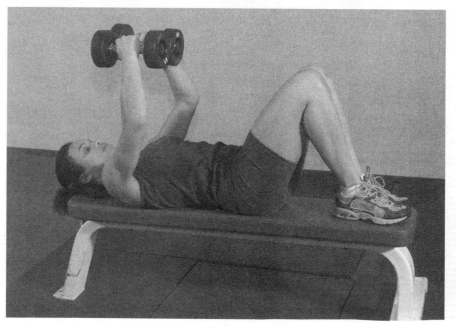

**Dumbbell Flye**

NOTE: This exercise can also be done on a common machine, often called a "pec deck." Sit on a bench and bend your arms at the elbow in front of you, with your forearms in a vertical position. Place your forearms against pads in front of your shoulders. Exhale and press against the pads together until they touch in front of your chest. Hold, then inhale and let the pads return to the starting position. Repeat.

### Dips

**Primary muscles used:** Chest
**Technique:** This exercises does not use weights—your body weight provides all the resistance. Find a set of "dip bars"—free-standing, parallel bars that are slightly wider than your shoulders and about chest high. Stand between the bars, rise up on your toes, and place your palms on top of the bars. Gently jump up and straighten your arms until your elbows lock. Your feet will be about a foot off the floor and your waist a few inches above the bars. Inhale and lower yourself gradually until your chest is in line with the bars. Bend your knees to keep your feet from touching the floor. Hold for a second, then exhale and push yourself back up until your elbows lock. Repeat.

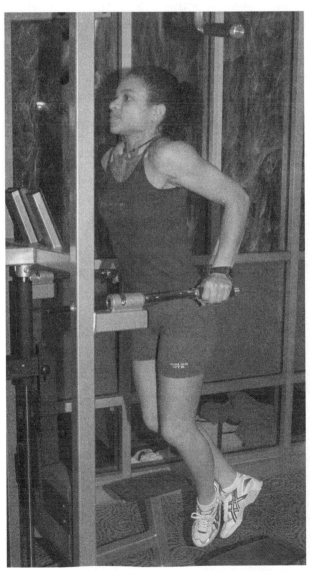
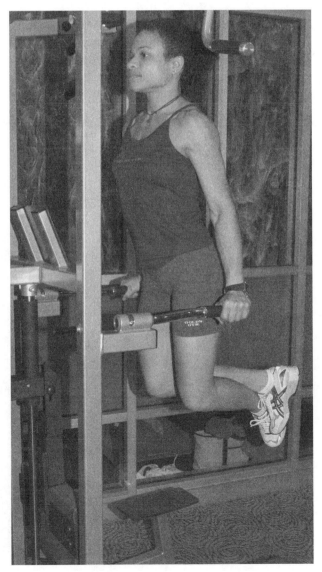

**Dips**

### Upright Row

*Primary muscles used:* Lats (back)

*Technique:* Stand with your feet slightly more than shoulder-width apart. Grab a barbell off the floor with an overhand grip (palms down, thumbs in) and your hands 8 to 10 inches apart. Let the bar rest against your thighs. Exhale and lift the bar straight up, keeping it close to your body, until it almost touches your chin. Keep your back straight and your legs straight as you lift. Hold the barbell under your chin for a second, then inhale and lower it to the starting position in front of your thighs. Repeat.

### Lat Pulldown

*Primary muscles used:* Lats (back)

*Technique:* This exercise is done on a machine that's found in almost every gym. It has a long horizontal bar over-head that's attached to a stack of weights by a cable. Kneel on the floor under the bar (or sit on a bench, if one is available). Extend your arms over-head and grab the bar with an over-hand grip and your hands 2 to 3 inches from the ends. Exhale as you pull the bar down smoothly in front of your face until it touches your chest. Hold for a second, then inhale and gradually let the bar return to the starting posi-tion. Repeat.

### Lateral Raise

*Primary muscles used:* Shoulders

*Technique:* Stand and hold a dumb-bell on each side of your body. Lean forward at the waist slightly, and bend your elbows a little. Exhale and slowly raise your arms, keeping them in line with your shoulders. Stop when the dumbbells are slightly higher than your shoulders. Don't let your body rock—this reduces the benefit to your shoulders. Hold the dumbbells at the topmost point for a second, then inhale and slowly lower them to your side. Repeat.

### Military Press

*Primary muscles used:* Shoulders

*Technique:* This exercise can be done with a barbell or on a machine.

*If you use a barbell:* Grab a barbell off the floor with an overhand grip and your hands placed slightly more than shoulder-width apart. Stand with the barbell against your thighs. Then hoist the barbell until it touches the top of your chest. (Your palms are underneath the bar for support.) Exhale and lift the barbell over your head until your elbows lock. Keep your legs stationary. Hold for a second, then gradually lower the barbell until it rests against your chest again. Start the next rep from your chest.

*If you use a machine:* Sit on a bench and grab the handle that's about even with your shoulders and connected

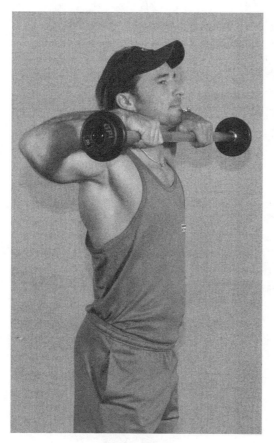

**Upright Row**

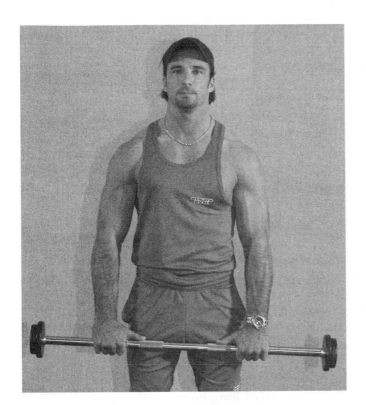

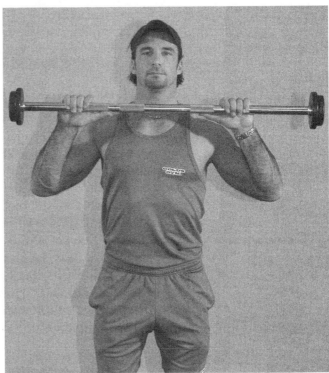

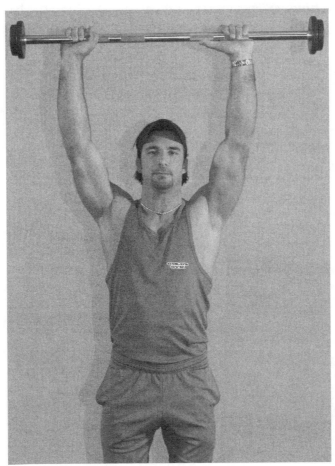

**Military Press**

to a weight stack. Press up on the handle, lifting the weight, until your elbows lock. Hold for a moment, then lower the handle until there is no resistance. Repeat.

### Arms

#### Curls

*Primary muscles used:* Biceps

*Technique:* Grab a barbell with an underhand grip (palms up, thumbs out) and your hands about shoulder-width apart. Stand and let the barbell rest against your thighs. Keeping your elbows close to your sides, exhale and raise the bar to your chest. Hold for a moment, then inhale and lower the bar to your thighs. Keep your elbows and upper arms stationary. Repeat.

#### Preacher Curl

*Primary muscles used:* Biceps

*Technique:* This exercise uses a "preacher bench," which has a small seat and an armrest platform about chest high that slopes down and away from the seat. Sit on the seat and place the backs of your upper arms on the sloping platform. Stretch your arms and grab a barbell with an underhand grip. Exhale and bend your arms, slowly bringing the barbell to the top of the platform (near your chin). Pause, then inhale and lower the barbell to the bottom of the platform, locking your elbows. Repeat.

NOTE: By not permitting use of your legs or upper body, this exercise isolates your biceps more than standing Curls.

#### Triceps Pushdown

*Primary muscles used:* Triceps

*Technique:* This exercise is similar to the Lat Pulldown described above. Stand in front of the machine, which has a long horizontal bar overhead. Grab the bar with an overhand grip and your hands 8 to 10 inches apart. Lower

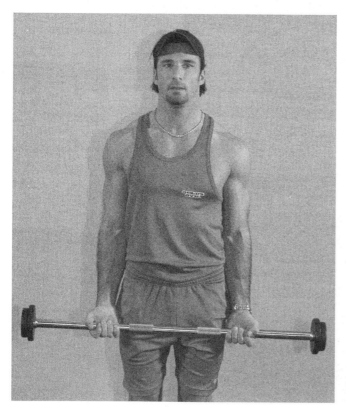
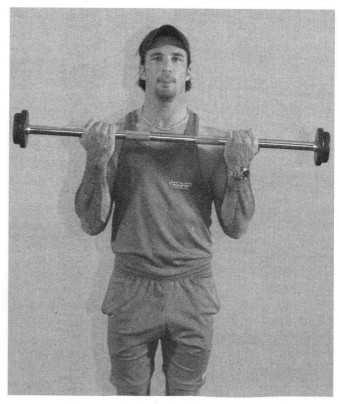

**Curls**

the bar until it's even with your chest. Tuck your elbows against your sides. Now exhale and press down on the bar with your upper arms *only*. Stop when the bar touches your thighs. Hold, then inhale and let the bar gradually rise to the starting position in front of your chest. Keep your upper arms against your sides. Repeat.

### Dips Behind Back

*Primary muscles used:* Triceps

*Technique:* This exercise is similar to parallel bar Dips, described above. No weights are used. Place two regular flat benches parallel to each other and about 4 to 5 feet apart. Place your heels on one bench and your palms on the other bench. Your buttocks will be suspended in the air, just in front of the rear bench. Your body will be in an L shape—legs parallel to the floor and torso at a 90-degree angle. Inhale, bend your arms at the elbow and carefully lower your buttocks until they almost touch the floor. Keep your heels on the front bench. Hold your body as low as possible for a second, then exhale and raise your body to the starting position, locking your elbows. Repeat.

### Dumbbell Wrist Curl

*Primary muscles used:* Forearms

*Technique:* Sit on a regular flat bench. Grab a dumbbell in one hand with an underhand grip. Lean forward and place your forearm on your thigh, with your wrist just beyond your knee. Lower your wrist toward the floor, letting the dumbbell roll toward the ends of your fingers. Then bend your wrist back toward your body, letting the dumbbell roll onto your palm. Repeat. Feel your forearm muscles stretch. Repeat with your opposite arm.

### Reverse Curl (illustrated on p. 30)

*Primary muscles used:* Forearms

*Technique:* Grab a barbell with an overhand grip and your hands placed about shoulder-width apart. Stand with the barbell in front of your thighs and elbows against your sides—this is the starting position. Exhale and raise your forearms *only* until the backs of your

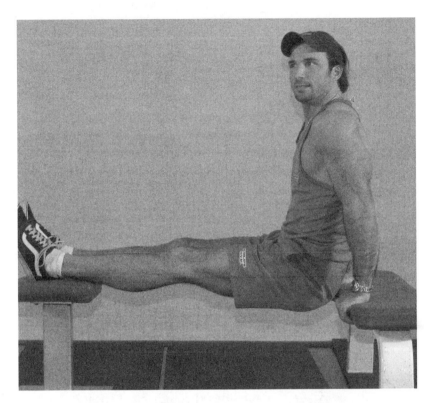

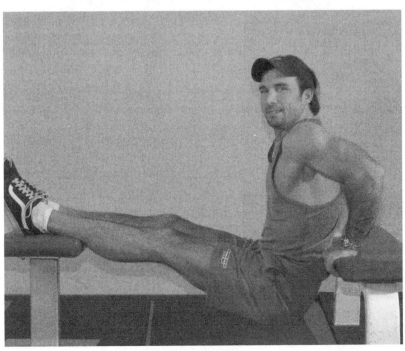

**Dips Behind Back**

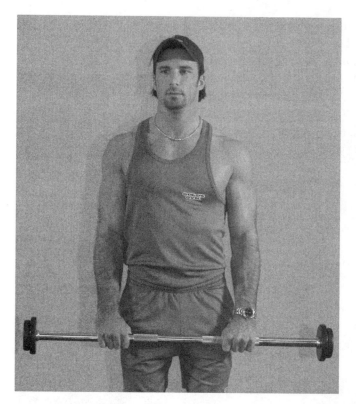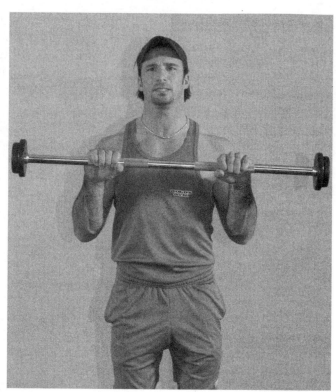

**Reverse Curl**

hands almost touch your chest. Hold, then inhale and lower the barbell to your thighs. Keep your upper arms at your sides throughout. Repeat.

### Legs

### Leg Extension

   **Primary muscles used:** Thighs
   **Technique:** This exercise uses a machine with a flat bench and two cylinder-shaped pads attached to a weight stack. Sit on the end of the bench with your legs hanging straight down from your knees. Place your shins against the backs of the pads. Grab the sides of the bench (or handles if it has them) and lift your legs straight up, raising the weight stack. Stop when your knees lock. Hold, then inhale and lower the pads to the starting position. Repeat.

### Squats

   **Primary muscles used:** Thighs
   **Technique:** Begin with a barbell resting on a rack at about shoulder height. Stand with your back to the bar, bend your knees slightly, and let the bar touch the back of your shoulders. Grab it with an overhand grip and your hands placed slightly more than shoulder-width apart. Carefully lift the bar off the rack. Make sure you have a good grip and stable footing. Place the bar against the back of your shoulders, then inhale and bend your knees until your thighs are parallel to the floor. Hold, then exhale and slowly rise, straightening your legs until you reach the starting position. Repeat.

   NOTE: This exercise can be dangerous if done improperly. As you lower yourself, keep the bar directly above your ankles; don't let the weight get too far in front of or behind your body, or you may lose your balance. Also, keep your head up and your eyes looking forward. This ensures that your thighs, not your back, bear most of the weight.

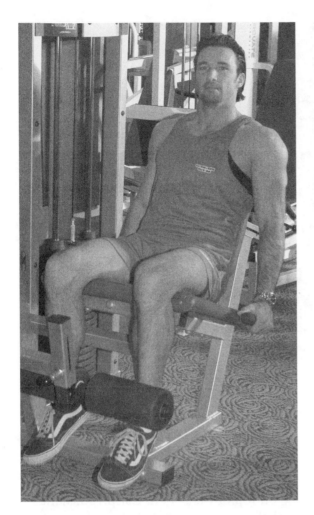
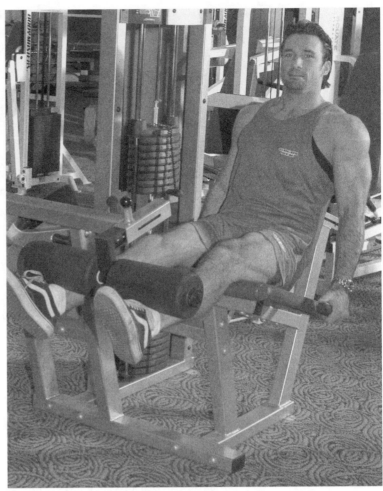

**Leg Extension**

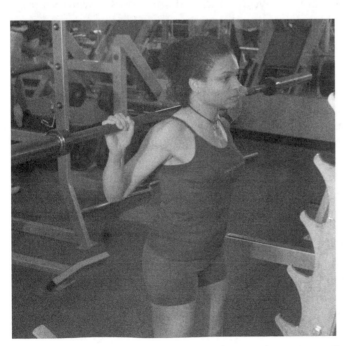
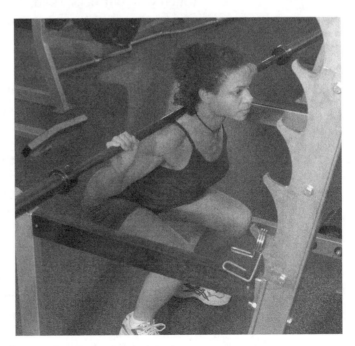

**Squats**

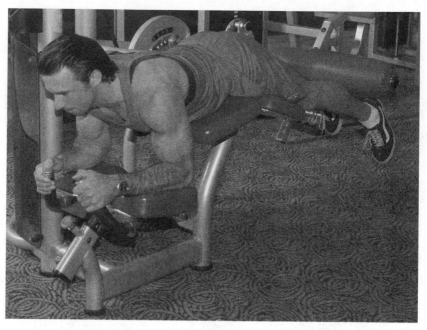

Leg Curl

### Leg Curl

*Primary muscles used:* Hamstrings

*Technique:* This exercise is done on a machine with a flat or inverted-V bench. Lie face down on the bench, and place your ankles under two cylinder-shaped pads. Bend your knees, then exhale and lift your lower legs until your feet almost touch your buttocks. Hold, then inhale and let the weights return your ankles to the starting position. Repeat.

### Calf Raise

*Primary muscles used:* Calves

*Technique:* This exercise starts out like Squats, described above. Stand with your back to a barbell that's resting on a shoulder-height rack. Grab the bar with an overhand grip and your hands placed slightly more than shoulder-width apart. Remove the bar from the rack and carefully place it on top of your shoulders. Position the balls of your feet on a block that's about 2 inches high, with your heels extended over the edge of the block. Exhale and raise your heels as high as possible, while keeping the barbell securely on your shoulders. Hold, then inhale and lower your heels to the floor. Repeat.

### Abs
### Crunches

*Primary muscles used:* Abs

*Technique:* Lie on your back on the floor in front of a flat bench. Bend your knees and place the backs of your calves on top of the bench. Clasp your hands behind your head. Exhale and raise your head and shoulders toward your knees, keeping your back on the floor. Inhale and lower yourself to the floor. Repeat.

NOTE: This is a very short movement. It's critical to do it slowly and deliberately to get the full effect.

### Leg Lifts (illustrated on p. 34)

*Primary muscles used:* Abs

*Technique:* Lie on your back on a flat bench with your buttocks at one end and your legs hanging loosely. Straighten your legs until they are parallel to the floor and even with the top of the bench. Grab the sides of the bench for support. Keeping your legs together and straight, exhale and raise them overhead until they are perpendicular to the floor. Pause, then slowly lower them to the starting position. Repeat.

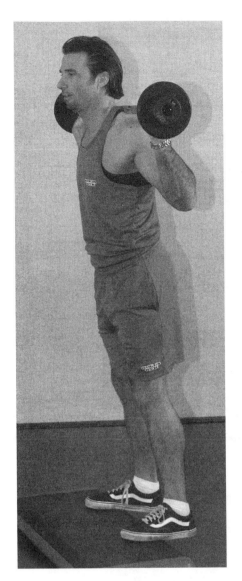
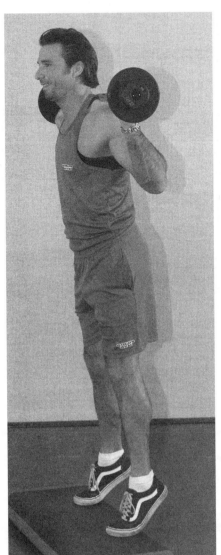
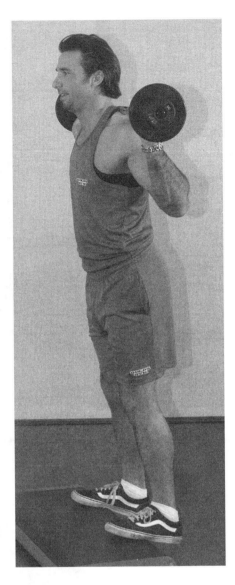

**Calf Raise**

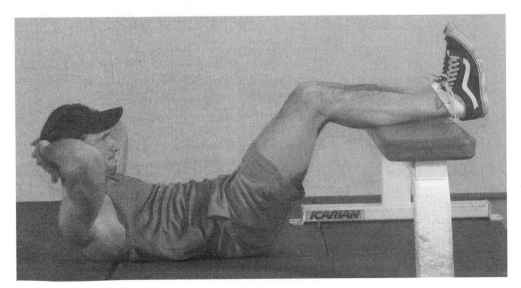

**Crunches**

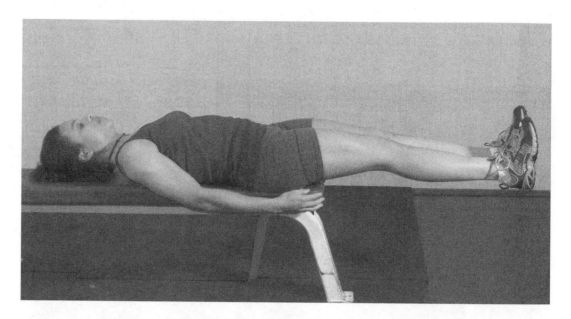

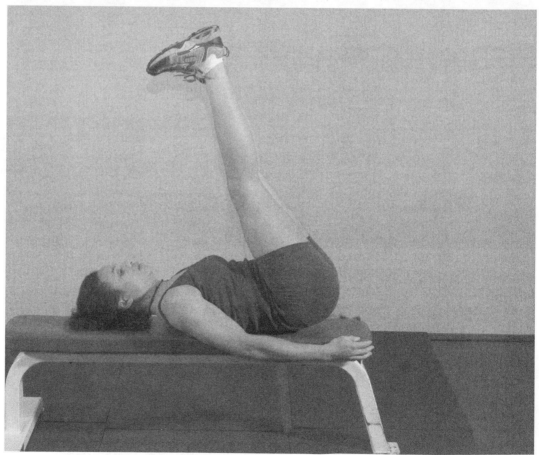

**Leg Lifts**

**3**

# Nutrition

"I hate to see misled people work hard in the gym, only to have their results ruined by eating the wrong foods."

—John Parillo, nutrition and training expert

When people think of bodybuilding, they consider weight training the key component, but nutrition is almost as important in achieving the physique you want.

If you eat junk food, all the weight lifting in the world won't produce a top-notch body. In recent years, we've learned a great deal about the importance of nutrition. Sure, we all slip up and eat things we shouldn't, and bodybuilders are no exception. It's not as if you can never cheat again if you're going to be a successful bodybuilder, but a major part of your training must be watching what you eat.

Just as you need to understand your muscles and how they work, you need to be aware of the basics of nutrition: protein, carbohydrates ("carbs"), and fat. Each plays a critical role in your diet. What do we mean by "diet"? To many people, "diet" means counting calories and starving themselves. That form of dieting is normally counterproductive. You may limit calories enough to lose weight for a short while, but almost invariably you gain it back.

In bodybuilding, "diet" simply means your overall eating habits. To add muscle, you have to consume a lot of calories. You can't get huge by eating like a bird.

"Train big, eat big, sleep big"— that's the advice some people give.

Naturally, *what* you eat is critical. For instance, if you take in too much fat, you won't achieve outstanding muscle definition. Bodybuilders face the delicate balance of eating enough to gain muscle mass but keeping their body fat percentage low enough for definition (about 8% to 11% for men and 7% to 9% for women).

There's no single perfect diet for everyone, just as there's no perfect weight training regimen for everyone. As you learn about nutrition, you'll be able to craft an eating plan that helps you achieve your fitness objectives. Knowledge is power—both in weight lifting and in eating. The two go hand in hand.

In the past, most people considered three square meals a day as the best diet. Nutritionists have learned that eating fewer, smaller meals each day

### DEVELOPING AN EATING PLAN

"Keeping a daily food record is crucial to sustained growth, since it enables you to accurately track how well you are keeping up with your dietary plan. The information gathered in your eating record provides the actual daily nutrient numbers, which will be critical for achieving your bodybuilding goals, especially in competition. . . .

"To grow, you must stress the muscles through training and eat sufficient food to provide the materials for recovery. . . .

"It is important to increase the amount of food you eat during the mid-morning, mid-afternoon, and post-training times. Of greatest importance is the post-training meal. During this time, your body is primed from the stress of the workout to literally soak up as would a sponge the proteins and carbohydrates that arrive into circulation."

—from *Gold's Gym Building Bulk*

is far better. Our bodies need to be fed often, but they don't need to be overwhelmed by large quantities. For instance, it's not good to eat a big meal of meat, vegetables, bread, and dessert an hour or so before bed. Those calories don't have time to be burned, and they'll transform into fat as you sleep.

Bodybuilders normally eat their largest meals during the day, when they're more active, rather than at night. They often prepare food in advance and take it with them so they can stick to their eating plan. You should do the same. By preparing meals in advance, you ensure that you have plenty of nutritious food on hand, and you won't be tempted to eat junk food.

Now let's focus on the three basic macronutrients: protein, carbs, and fat.

## PROTEIN

Of the three macronutrients, protein is the most critical for bodybuilders. Protein is responsible for growth, maintenance, and repair of muscle tissue, which is why top bodybuilders constantly monitor their protein intake.

In general, a bodybuilder needs twice as much protein as the average person. The best sources of protein are eggs, fish, poultry, meat, and dairy products—the animal proteins. Plant proteins—from foods like rice, beans, corn, peas, and nuts—are not as easily assimilated into the body as animal proteins.

Few top bodybuilders are vegetarian. However, one of the most famous bodybuilders of all time, Bill Pearl, has been a vegetarian for decades. He was a champion bodybuilder in the 1950s and '60s and has since written best-selling fitness books. He says that he lowered his blood pressure and cholesterol and eliminated many aches and pains by cutting out meat. "With each succeeding year on the diet, I've felt better," Pearl says. "I'm healthier, and I can train with more energy."

A longtime friend of Pearl's, Arnold Schwarzenegger, says he respects Pearl's decision not to eat meat: "Bill never talked me into becoming a vegetarian, but he did convince me that a vegetarian could become a champion bodybuilder."

Like most elite bodybuilders, Schwarzenegger believes that meat is too beneficial to give up. Meat is a complete protein, that is, it contains all the amino acids—the building blocks of protein. By contrast, vegetables, nuts, and fruits lack one or more of the essential amino acids and are considered incomplete proteins. Therefore, a person would have to eat a wide range and larger amounts of plant protein foods to get the same benefit that a small serving of meat would provide.

Mike Matarazzo, one of today's top bodybuilders, says he eats three to four pounds of meat every day. "I load up my freezer with beef and chicken," Matarazzo says.

Some nutritional experts say that it's possible to eat too much protein and that excessive amounts can damage the liver and kidneys. Most top bodybuilders, however, believe it's safe—and necessary—to consume a lot of protein.

The U.S. government recommends that the average person eat 0.36 grams of protein every day for each pound of body weight. For a 180-pound man, that's about 65 grams of protein per day. If that person is a bodybuilder, conventional bodybuilding wisdom says that he or she should consume twice that, because it's believed that too little protein will lead to greater muscle soreness and fatigue after a workout.

### Protein Supplements

Unlike some nutrients, protein cannot be stored in the body. Instead, it must be taken in continually to be useful—this is another reason to eat frequently. In order to get enough protein, most bodybuilders take protein supplements, usually in powder form and mixed with juice, milk, or water.

Most of today's supplements have little or no fat and taste much better than the supplements of the past. You don't have to hold your nose to force down a protein drink anymore. Protein supplements are handy because they're much easier to prepare and consume than a full meal—while providing most of the same nutrients.

Cost, however, can be a significant factor, so be sure to compare prices on supplements. Some are extraordinarily expensive, while other, much cheaper supplements are just as beneficial.

Protein supplements are usually made from whey, egg whites, soy, or milk. There are differing views on which protein source is best. Some medical researchers, for instance, say that soy protein can help lower cholesterol in some people. If you have a problem with cholesterol, you may want to consider a soy-based supplement.

A very basic, cheap protein supplement that's been around for years is powdered milk. It can be mixed with water or milk or perhaps blended with yogurt to produce an inexpensive protein supplement. It won't have all the benefits of today's high-tech supplements, which are packed with vitamins and minerals, but it does provide top-quality protein to enhance muscle growth.

## CARBOHYDRATES

Carbohydrates are the body's main source of energy. Although protein and fat supply some energy, about 50% of a bodybuilder's calories should come from carbohydrates.

Carbs fall into two categories: *simple* and *complex*.

Simple carbs provide a quick burst of energy. When they are digested, they turn into glucose, a major source of energy that can be burned rapidly. Candy is one example of a simple carb; fruit is another, healthier type.

Complex carbs, on the other hand, fuel the body over a longer period of time. Everyone needs both types of carbohydrates, but bodybuilders should focus on complex carbs because they provide a more sustained energy supply throughout the day.

Complex carbohydrates are broken down further into *fibrous* and *starchy* carbs. Sources of fibrous carbs include asparagus, green beans, broccoli, lettuce, mushrooms, spinach, and zucchini. Examples of sources of starchy carbs are red beans, corn, oatmeal, peas, pasta, potatoes, rice, and tomatoes.

## GLYCEMIC INDEX (GI) FOR COMMON FOODS

| Food | GI | Food | GI | Food | GI | Food | GI |
|---|---|---|---|---|---|---|---|
| Peanuts | 13 | Sausage | 28 | Rye bread | 42 | White bread | 69 |
| Soybeans | 16 | Lentils | 29 | Grapes | 45 | White rice | 70 |
| Fructose | 20 | Kidney beans | 29 | Oatmeal | 49 | Whole wheat bread | 72 |
| Cherries | 23 | Skim milk | 32 | White spaghetti | 50 | Honey | 87 |
| Plums | 25 | Whole milk | 34 | Sweet potatoes | 51 | Carrots | 92 |
| Grapefruit | 26 | Pears | 34 | Potato chips | 51 | Russet potato | 98 |
| Peaches | 26 | Yogurt | 36 | Corn | 59 | Glucose | 100 |
| | | Ice cream | 36 | Banana | 62 | | |
| | | Tomatoes | 38 | Beets | 64 | | |
| | | Apples | 39 | Raisins | 64 | | |

A measurement called a glycemic index (GI) has been developed in recent years to indicate how quickly your body consumes a carbohydrate. Foods with a high GI produce a large, sudden release of glucose—and energy. Those with a low GI are used slowly, over a long period of time, and help ensure a steady blood sugar level throughout the day.

## Low-Carb Diets

In today's weight-conscious world, people are constantly looking for a diet that can produce quick weight loss. Over the past few years, low-carb diets have become extremely popular. For some people, they can be very effective. Here's how they work: When fewer carbs are available, the body burns more fat for energy, thereby leading to weight loss.

A low-carb diet may sound appealing, but it can have serious drawbacks. First, lowering your carbohydrate intake can reduce your energy level and lead to dehydration. Second, as your body burns fat, it may also burn muscle. In other words, you can lose some of the muscle mass you've worked so hard to attain. Third, carbohydrates are necessary for proper functioning of your brain, heart, and vital organs.

As you can see, carbs are vital to a person's well-being. Be very careful with eating plans that recommend low amounts of carbohydrates.

## Carbohydrate Supplements

Because it can be difficult to get enough quality carbs in a regular diet, carb supplements are popular with many of today's top bodybuilders. Since an intense workout burns a tremendous amount of carbohydrates, some people say that you should eat 50 to 75 grams of carbs within 20 minutes of finishing your workout or your body may burn protein instead; that, in turn, can hinder muscle growth.

Some everyday foods, such as carrot juice, are extremely high in carbohydrates. Graham crackers and honey are also good. Eating these foods can be an excellent way to add quality carbs without taking a high-priced carb supplement.

## FAT

Of all the macronutrients, fat has the worst reputation. People hear the word "fat" and think obesity, but fat plays a vital role in a well-balanced diet.

It should comprise about 10% to 15% of your food intake.

Fat is a secondary source of energy, but it has twice as many calories per gram as protein or carbohydrates. It's easy to understand why people gain weight by eating too much fat.

In addition to providing energy, fat cushions and protects the major organs and insulates the body against extreme cold. It also helps maintain healthy skin and hair and transports vitamins A, D, E, and K throughout our bodies.

There are three different types of fat: *saturated, unsaturated,* and *polyunsaturated.*

Saturated fat is found primarily in animal products such as beef, lamb, pork, butter, and most cheeses. Saturated fat has been linked to high cholesterol levels and an increased risk of heart disease. Foods high in saturated fat often taste good, but your diet should not include large amounts of this type of fat.

Foods high in unsaturated fat include avocados, cashews, peanuts and peanut butter, and olives and olive oil. This type of fat is preferable to saturated fat.

The third type, polyunsaturated fat, is present in almonds, pecans, walnuts, most margarine, mayonnaise, and soybean oil. Medical research has shown that some people who eat large amounts of polyunsaturated fat along with small amounts of saturated fat have lower cholesterol levels than others.

## WATER

Water is also one of the basic nutrients, and people often overlook its importance. Water offers many benefits. It's essential for proper digestion, removes waste from the body, and regulates body temperature. As an illustration of water's importance, people can live for weeks without food, but for only a few days without water.

Muscles are composed of 72% water by weight. Therefore, as you sweat during exercise, you're losing muscle mass.

You should keep a water bottle with you during workouts and take frequent sips. Try to drink *before* you become thirsty. Many experts say that everyone should drink eight 8-ounce glasses of water a day, and bodybuilders need to drink even more. Other liquids such as juice, soft drinks, and coffee do not count toward your water intake.

Some bodybuilders make the mistake of trying to purge water from their bodies before a contest by using diuretics. They think that excess water beneath the skin reduces muscle definition. However, diuretics can be extremely dangerous, or even fatal. Don't deprive your body of water.

## VITAMINS

"Take your vitamins." That's advice many of our moms gave us while growing up, and they were right.

Vitamins are organic substances that contribute to many important bodily functions. We all need specific vitamins in certain amounts for optimum health. However, most nutritional experts believe that no one—not even a bodybuilder—needs vitamins in massive amounts. Some people take huge doses of Vitamin C to try to prevent colds, but this is generally not considered beneficial, and the result is simply high-priced urine.

Vitamins fall into two categories: *water soluble* and *fat soluble.*

Water-soluble vitamins cannot be stored in the body, and excess amounts are eliminated in urine. Because they can't be retained, water-soluble vita-

## KEY VITAMINS—THEIR SOURCES AND FUNCTIONS

### WATER-SOLUBLE VITAMINS

**Vitamin $B_1$ (thiamin)**

*Sources:* Nuts, whole grains, dried beans, peas, pork

*Functions:* Helps with carbohydrate metabolism and functioning of the nervous system; improves muscle tone; reduces fatigue

**Vitamin $B_2$ (riboflavin)**

*Sources:* Eggs, milk, beef, poultry, liver, asparagus, peanuts

*Functions:* Is necessary for normal cell growth; helps with metabolism of carbohydrates, fat, and protein; promotes good vision and healthy hair, skin, and nails

**Vitamin $B_3$ (niacin)**

*Sources:* Fish, poultry, green leafy vegetables, dried fruit, whole grains, milk, eggs

*Functions:* Stimulates circulation and digestion; helps maintain healthy skin

**Vitamin $B_{12}$ (cyanocobalamin)**

*Sources:* Meat, poultry, cheese, milk, eggs, yogurt, oysters

*Functions:* Is necessary for development of red blood cells; helps with functioning of the nervous system; promotes metabolism of protein, carbohydrates, and fat

**Vitamin C (ascorbic acid)**

*Sources:* Citrus fruits, berries, green leafy vegetables, potatoes, tomatoes, green peppers

*Functions:* Helps build connective tissue in skin, cartilage, and bones; strengthens the immune system; improves absorption of iron; allows wounds to heal more quickly

### FAT-SOLUBLE VITAMINS

**Vitamin A (retinol)**

*Sources:* Carrots, yellow and green vegetables, fish, fruits, milk, butter

*Functions:* Is necessary for normal growth and tissue repair; improves night vision; fights bacteria and infection; promotes healthy skin, hair, and membranes

**Vitamin D (cholecalciferol)**

*Sources:* Tuna, salmon, cod liver oil, egg yolk, whole milk

*Functions:* Improves absorption of calcium and phosphorus for healthy bones; maintains functioning of the nervous system and the heart. NOTE: Sunlight manufactures Vitamin D when it comes in contact with skin.

**Vitamin E (alpha-tocopherol)**

*Sources:* Nuts, whole grain products, green leafy vegetables, fish, wheat germ, vegetable oils

*Functions:* Promotes healthy cell membranes; helps prevent blood clots

**Vitamin K (menadione)**

*Sources:* Cheddar cheese, spinach, cabbage, cauliflower, liver

*Function:* Is necessary for blood clotting

---

mins need to be taken daily if you don't get enough of them in the food you eat. Some important water-soluble vitamins include $B_1$ (thiamin), $B_2$ (riboflavin), $B_3$ (niacin), $B_{12}$ (cyanocobalamin), biotin, and Vitamin C (ascorbic acid).

Fat-soluble vitamins, unlike water-soluble ones, can be stored. They can therefore be taken less often. Important fat-soluble vitamins are A, D, E, and K.

Many experts believe that food loses much of its vitamin content through processing and the addition of preservatives. Unfortunately, much of the food we eat today is highly processed, making it difficult to get enough vitamins through diet alone. Bodybuilders, because of their intense workouts,

definitely need to take a basic vitamin supplement, which can provide good insurance against vitamin deficiency. Follow the dosage suggestions on the bottle unless advised to do otherwise by your doctor.

## MINERALS

Unlike vitamins, minerals are inorganic substances. They promote the growth, maintenance, and repair of tissue. Minerals also assist in muscle contraction and the functioning of the nervous system. Some common minerals are calcium, magnesium, and potassium.

Like vitamins, minerals are needed in relatively small amounts. A well-

## KEY MINERALS—THEIR SOURCES AND FUNCTIONS

### Calcium
*Sources:* Milk, egg yolk, green leafy vegetables, clams, oysters
*Functions:* Helps develop strong teeth and bones; prevents muscle cramping; promotes normal blood clotting and heart function

### Phosphorus
*Sources:* Meat, fish, poultry, nuts, whole grain cereals, beans
*Functions:* Assists in muscle contraction, nerve function, and bone and tooth formation

### Magnesium
*Sources:* Nuts, fish, wheat germ, green leafy vegetables, whole grain cereals
*Functions:* Is necessary for muscle and nerve activity; helps with bone formation

### Potassium
*Sources:* Fruits, milk, beans, meat, cereals
*Functions:* Helps with metabolism of protein and carbohydrates; aids in functioning of the heart, nervous system, and kidneys

### Sodium
*Sources:* Table salt, milk, eggs, seafood
*Functions:* Helps regulate body fluids; assists in muscle contraction

### Chlorine
*Sources:* Table salt, seafood, milk, eggs, meat
*Function:* Promotes proper pH balance in the blood

---

balanced diet may provide all the minerals you need, but it's wise to take a mineral supplement to prevent deficiency. "No athlete should go without a multivitamin/mineral supplement," says Lee Labrada, two-time Mr. Olympia runner-up.

However, there's no need to take massive doses. Six-time Mr. Olympia titlist Dorian Yates says vitamins and minerals should serve only a complementary role in your diet. "Supplementation is not nearly as important as eating a well-balanced and nutritious diet," he says.

## CALORIE CONSUMPTION

How many calories should you consume in a day? There's no single answer for everybody, but as a bodybuilder, you need more calories than a sedentary person in order to achieve muscle gain. How many more calories you need depends on your metabolism rate and on the intensity and frequency of your workouts.

Some people have a much higher metabolism than others, meaning that they burn many more calories than other people with the same activity level. Earlier in the book, we discussed the three main body types: *ectomorph* (naturally thin people), *endomorph* (naturally heavy people), and *mesomorph* (people with good natural physiques who gain muscle easily). Knowing your body type will help to determine how much you should eat. You may have to eat almost constantly in order to maintain muscle mass, or you may struggle to keep your weight down.

In general, the harder you train, the more calories you need. Top bodybuilders don't train at the same intensity year-round. It's impossible to do so—both mentally and physically. When a contest is far off, they scale back their workouts; when an event is approaching, they increase workout intensity. For each level they adjust their diet and calorie intake accordingly.

You should learn to be flexible in the number of calories you consume. For instance, if you're not getting to the gym often to work out, you need to reduce your food intake.

When a person stops lifting weight, muscle does not automatically turn

## WORDS TO TRAIN BY

"Start eating correctly when you begin your program. Diet is the key to losing weight. Remember, training and eating go hand in hand. I don't disagree with taking supplements or vitamins—as long as it's in moderation."

—Frank Sepe, top bodybuilder

to fat, thereby causing the person to become overweight. Former bodybuilders become overweight when they stop lifting weights *and* don't reduce their calorie intake. If your calorie intake matches your workout intensity, you shouldn't develop a weight problem.

Before you begin a serious weight training regimen, record your body weight and body fat percentage. The easiest, least expensive way to measure your body fat percentage is with a skinfold caliper, which resembles a pliers. You pinch your skin at certain places on your body and use the caliper to measure the thickness of the pinched skin. A more accurate body fat test, in which you're submerged in water, may be arranged through a physician or trainer.

Start keeping a daily log of what you eat, including the number of calories and the amount of protein, carbohydrates, and fat. This will establish a baseline if you need to change your eating habits later.

Don't automatically increase or decrease your calorie intake at the beginning. Start your workout program, continue eating as you normally would, and then see if you gain or lose weight. If you're losing weight (and you don't want to), you can afford to take in more calories.

On the other hand, you may find that you're not losing weight even with intense workouts. Because muscle weighs more than fat, it's possible—even common—to add muscle and lose fat without dropping weight. Body weight alone is not a complete measure of your fitness. However, you may find that you still need to cut calories in order to achieve your desired weight.

There's no need to become fanatical about calorie intake—that is, count the calories in every cracker or slice of bread. That can be counterproductive and lead to binge eating because you've been starving yourself. As you become more experienced in bodybuilding, you'll be able to feel when your body needs food and trust your appetite. Bodybuilders must learn to personalize their eating habits and calorie intake just as they fine-tune their workout regimens.

## MEAL FREQUENCY AND SELECTION

In recent years, bodybuilders and nutritional experts have stressed the importance of frequent, smaller meals. Our bodies need to be fed more than three times a day, particularly if we're engaged in heavy weight training. When we eat less at each meal, our bodies can digest the food more easily and we don't wind up feeling "stuffed" and lethargic.

As a rule of thumb, you should eat five or six times a day—or about every two to three hours. By following this pattern, you'll never get so hungry that you're tempted to overeat or to eat junk food.

The key to successful meal frequency is planning—developing the discipline to decide what to eat a few days in advance so that meals mesh with training and fitness objectives.

Few of us can arrange to eat five or six meals at home every day, so it's important to learn to set aside time to prepare and package food to take along—perhaps a chicken breast or some brown rice to eat at work. The meals you prepare can be small enough to be eaten quickly. By eating a small meal every few hours, you'll maintain your energy level better than if you were eating two or three large meals a day.

If you have to eat at restaurants, you can still maintain a healthy eating plan if you carefully read menus and check the ingredients of menu items. These days, restaurants are accustomed to diners who watch what they eat. Ask the server for more details if necessary. It's not out of order to ask that an item be specially prepared if it's not on the menu.

Be smart when grocery shopping—read labels. Fortunately, most packaged foods have a detailed ingredients label so that it's easy to find out the number of calories per serving and the amount of protein, carbohydrates, and fat.

Pay attention to what you put in your body. You'll see the difference.

## GENERAL EATING GUIDELINES

Because of the almost infinite variety of food choices, it's difficult to provide sample menus that would suit everyone and meet each person's individual needs. Other books are devoted entirely to diet and food preparation for bodybuilders. Here we'll touch on some of the broad "dos" and "don'ts" of food selection and preparation.

- Pay attention to the ratio of carbohydrates, protein, and fat in your meals. Ideally, your diet should consist of about 50% carbs, 35% protein, and 15% fat.

- Choose fresh fruits and vegetables instead of canned or frozen ones. The latter often contain sugar, salt, and preservatives that can be harmful.
- Select fresh meats instead of processed meats (like lunch meat) for the same reason that you choose fresh fruits and vegetables.
- Eat white meat (such as chicken breasts) instead of dark meat (such as chicken thighs), because white meat has less fat. Remove the skin to further reduce the fat.
- Eat fish, which typically has even less fat than white meat. A popular choice for bodybuilders is tuna, which is inexpensive and easy to take with you, since it's canned and requires no refrigeration. Select tuna that's packed in spring water, not oil. Oil contains many useless calories.
- Broil or bake your meat, poultry, or fish. Never fry it.
- Don't overcook vegetables, because overcooking destroys many of the vitamins and minerals they contain.
- Buy low-fat or no-fat versions of dairy products like milk and yogurt.
- Use fewer egg yolks, because they're high in fat and cholesterol. You don't have to give them up entirely; if you fix three scrambled eggs, for example, you can include one yolk and toss out the other two.
- Choose whole grain breads, which have more fiber and are more nutritious than breads made with white, processed flour.
- Avoid toppings that are high in calories and fat. A dry baked potato is great, but a baked potato with butter and sour cream is not. Lettuce has almost no calories or fat until you add salad dressing, so be sure to pick a dressing that's low-fat or no-fat. When eating meats, avoid

**WORDS TO TRAIN BY**

"You can have the best diet in the world, but if you don't follow it, it does you no good."

—Flex Wheeler, Mr. Olympia runner-up

gravy. With pasta, stay away from sauces made with heavy cream.

- Pick fruit instead of candy if you want to eat sweets. Go easy on fruits and fruit juices, however, because even though they're healthier than candy and soft drinks, they're still rich in sugar and calories.
- Learn to discipline yourself so you don't succumb to impulsive eating. We all "fall off the wagon" sometimes and eat foods that aren't a part of our recommended diet. Just try to make sure that you do so only occasionally, and then resume your eating plan.
- Avoid fad diets recommending that you drastically cut back or eliminate major nutrients, such as carbohydrates.

- Don't try to shed more than 2 pounds a week if you want to lose weight.
- Add variety to your diet. Eat a wide range of healthy foods. The more you enjoy your food, the more likely you are to stick with good eating habits.
- Make wise use of the excellent meal-replacement products that are available, such as powders and drinks. If you're short on time, you can take them instead of preparing a meal. However, never rely on replacement products and supplements entirely; they can't take the place of healthy eating.
- Eat nuts and dried fruit for a quick snack, but in moderation.
- Always eat breakfast. Some people skip breakfast to try to cut calories, but that's not wise. You need a good supply of fuel to start your day. Otherwise, you may find yourself low on energy and be tempted to eat junk food.
- Wait at least one hour after eating to work out so that your food can be properly digested.

# 4

# Intermediate Chest Exercises

"I'm never dogmatic when it comes to my training regimen.
If I discover something new, I don't hesitate to use it."

—Flex Wheeler, Mr. Olympia runner-up

After a few months of weight training, you should know whether you want to pursue bodybuilding seriously. If you like your results, you're probably hooked. It's exciting to see your physique take shape and muscles appear that you didn't know existed.

When you decide to stay with bodybuilding, you need to tackle more advanced exercises. The basic exercises we described in Chapter 2 cover all the major muscle groups in your upper and lower body, and you can keep doing them and make progress. Even the best bodybuilders continue to do some of them.

Nevertheless, if you really want to excel and set yourself apart from others, you need to expand the variety of your weightlifting exercises. Your muscles can become accustomed to the same exercises if they're done repeatedly, and they will no longer respond as well.

You need to constantly introduce new exercises to your regimen. Some pros call this "shocking" the muscles. The purpose is to make a muscle perform a movement that's unfamiliar, and the result is new muscle growth. Different exercises attack different parts of the muscle. For instance, the Standing Barbell Curl works the biceps as effectively as any single exercise, but it concentrates on only part of the biceps. Like most muscles, the biceps is complex and contains several areas.

To achieve maximum development, you must do exercises that work all areas of a muscle. In this chapter and the ones that follow, we'll describe numerous specialized exercises to target certain muscle groups.

There's no need to perform all the intermediate exercises we'll describe, certainly not on a consistent basis. Instead, choose the exercises that best suit your body and your goals. Ideally, you'll rotate exercises: select a group that produces results, then switch to others later, and so on. Even the most dedicated bodybuilder in the world can get burned out by doing the same exercises over and over—and your muscles can go unchallenged. By introducing variety in your workout, you can increase your intensity and make greater gains.

## WORDS TO TRAIN BY

"The trick to bodybuilding is to put an overload on your muscles. The secret . . . is to push up a heavy weight with the isolated strength of the muscle you are trying to train."

—Arnold Schwarzenegger

Pay close attention to the description that accompanies each exercise. It's crucial to perform them with correct form to avoid injury and get the maximum benefit.

Before we focus on the intermediate chest exercises, we'll briefly describe the chest muscles. This will help you understand how the muscles work and will help you choose exercises that meet your needs.

## MUSCLES OF THE CHEST

All great bodybuilders have well-developed chests. The pectorals, or chest muscles, are so large and prominent that they can't be hidden.

A massive chest anchors the upper body and enhances the appearance of your shoulders, arms, and abs. When you see photos of Arnold Schwarzenegger, for instance, his chest grabs your eye. His pectorals, and those of other champs, look like thick slabs of sculpted granite.

Compared to some other muscles, chest muscles can be developed fairly easily. Most people enjoy working the chest, because they can easily see and feel the muscles as they lift and enjoy the pump.

Pectorals are fan-shaped and cover the upper rib cage, then extend across to the upper arms and up to the collarbone. In the simplest sense, pecs allow you to move your arms across your body. They have four distinct parts: upper, lower, inner, and outer. Each part must be fully developed, defined, and separate from the others to receive high marks in judging.

To illustrate the effect of different exercises on your chest muscles, let's single out Bench Press, one of the basic chest exercises. It's outstanding, but it works mainly the middle of the chest. However, if you do Bench Press on an incline or decline bench, you shift the focus to the upper or lower pecs. An incline bench works the upper chest, a decline bench the lower. (Some benches are adjustable and can be made flat, as well as inclined and declined. Most gyms, however, have separate, dedicated flat benches, incline benches, and decline benches.)

If you don't have access to an incline or decline bench, you can achieve similar results with a flat bench. For instance, you can lower the barbell to your lower chest to develop the lower pecs and to your upper chest to work the upper pecs.

You can also change your hand position on the bar. Normally, you perform Bench Press with your hands slightly more than shoulder-width apart. If you widen your grip by a few inches, you shift effort to the outer pecs. The reverse is also true: If you bring your hands closer together, you work the inner pecs more.

Chest exercises fall into two main categories: *presses* and *flyes*. Presses involve lifting a barbell or dumbbell vertically over your chest (or using a machine that performs the same movement). Flyes involve raising and lowering weights horizontally to the sides of your chest. They too can be done with free weights or machines. Presses primarily work the center of the pecs from top to bottom, while flyes generally target the outside and inside pecs.

You need to do a wide range of presses and flyes to get complete pectoral development. Some top bodybuilders have built tremendous chests with only a few exercises, but they are most likely genetically predisposed to having large chest muscles. For most people, variety is critical to good progress.

Here are some key points to keep in mind when doing chest exercises:

- **Be careful.** Have a spotter or someone at your side when you use free weights. It's easy to become overconfident in your strength and grab a barbell with too much weight. You may wind up with the barbell on your chest and be unable to move it. That can be scary, as well as embarrassing. You can yell for help and someone will come to your aid, but it's much more reassuring to have a spotter standing by. Besides helping you if you get in trouble, he or she can assist you with a final rep or two after you become fatigued. It's these last few reps, even if assisted, that often produce the greatest results.
- **Warm up.** A strained chest muscle can put you out of action for weeks. It can be painful and slow to heal. With a proper warm-up, fortunately, a strained muscle is easy to avoid. This involves doing at least one set with light weight and more reps than you normally would. A warm-up set loosens your muscles and lets them get the feel of the exercise movement before you move up to heavy weight. A warm-up set can also prepare you mentally.
- **Barbells, dumbbells, and cables produce slightly different results.** With barbells, it's possible to use heavy weight to develop greater mass and strength. With dumbbells, you can't use as much weight because you're only lifting with one arm at a time. However, dumbbells allow you a greater range of motion than

barbells, which can be essential in some exercises. Cables attached to weight stacks are common devices on machines. Like dumbbells, cables provide a wide range of movement. They also allow for a smooth, safe lifting motion.
- **Keep your chest development in proportion to the rest of your body.** Some bodybuilders get fixated on having a huge chest. They do Bench Press over and over, at the expense of exercises for other muscles. The result is an unbalanced physique. It looks somewhat ridiculous to have a bowed-out chest and bird-like arms and legs.

**WORDS TO TRAIN BY**

"Although my arms and calves responded fairly quickly when I started training, my chest was pitifully weak with no peak muscle to speak of. I used to dream of having massive bulbous pecs like those of Arnold."

—Dorian Yates, six-time Mr. Olympia

## EXERCISES

### Upper Pecs

*Incline Press* (illustrated on pp. 48–49)

*Technique:* This is identical to Bench Press, described in Chapter 2, except that you lie on an incline bench instead of a flat one. Place your feet on the floor at the end of the bench. With an overhand grip, grab the barbell that's resting on supports above your head, placing your hands slightly more than shoulder-width apart. Raise the bar straight up until it's off the supports. Bring the bar forward until it's directly over your chest, then slowly lower it until the bar touches your

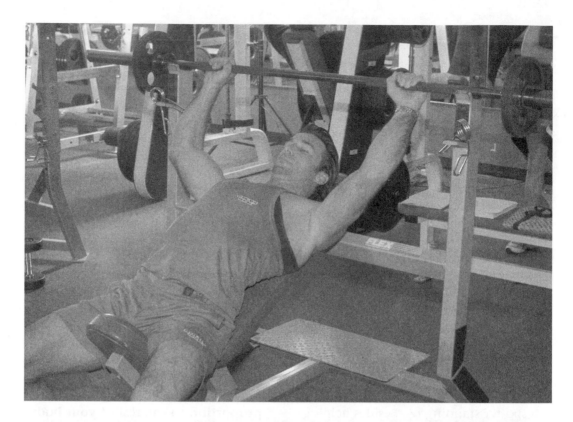

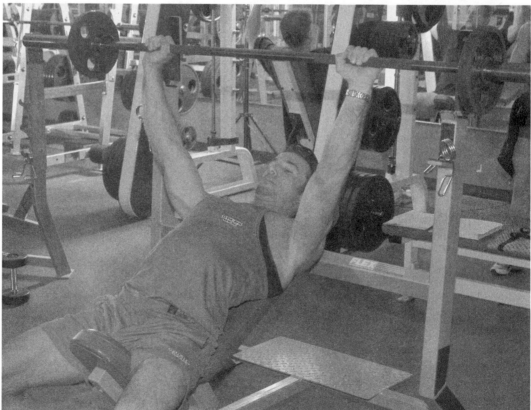

Incline Press ...

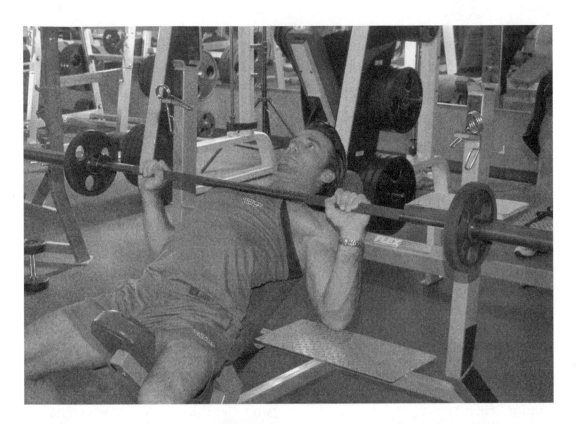

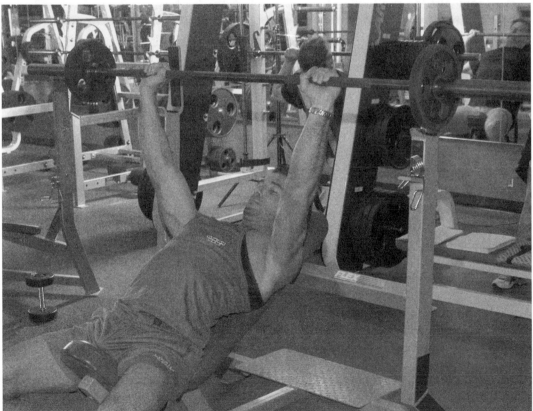

... Incline Press

chest. Don't let it bounce off your body. Keep your elbows close to your sides and slightly behind your torso to achieve maximum range of motion. Pause when the bar touches your chest, then lift it straight up, locking your elbows. Repeat.

NOTE: Be sure to keep the weight securely balanced during this exercise. When you bench press on an incline bench, the barbell will have a different balance point than when you bench press on a flat bench. Don't let the weight drift back over your head or forward over your abdomen. Use light weight at first until you're sure you can lift and lower the weight smoothly and under control. It's a good idea to have a spotter at first. Incline Press is a tremendous exercise for upper chest development, but you probably won't be able to use as much weight as you can for Bench Press.

You may also do the Incline Press with dumbbells, which allow a slightly longer range of motion than a barbell does. With dumbbells, you start with your palms toward each other, then twist your wrists 90 degrees as you lift so that the palms are oriented toward your feet at the top.

### Incline Flye

*Technique:* This is identical to the Dumbbell Flye, described in Chapter 2, except that you lie on an incline bench. With your hands at your sides, hold a dumbbell in each hand, even with the top of the bench. Extend your arms to the side until your elbows are only slightly bent. Raise the dumbbells upward on a wide path until they are directly over your chest, similar to a hugging motion. Let them touch briefly, then pause. Make sure you have a secure grip, then lower the dumbbells along the same path until they are again even with the top of the bench. Keep your arms bent slightly at the elbow throughout. Repeat.

NOTE: As with the Incline Press, it will take a few sets to get the "feel" of the Incline Flye versus the Dumbbell Flye. Use light weight until you can completely control the dumbbells. Keep them in line over your chest throughout the movement; don't let your arms drift backward so that the dumbbells are over your head or forward so that they are over your abdomen. Your palms should be oriented toward each other throughout the exercise. As with the Dumbbell Flye, don't lower the dumbbells too far to the side on the way down. They should not touch the floor, or you may strain your chest muscles; lower them only to the top of the bench.

### Low-Pulley Cable Crossover
(illustrated on p. 52)

*Technique:* Stand midway between two weight stacks, each of which has a pulley and cable attached. Place your feet slightly more than shoulder-width apart and bend your knees a little. Lean forward until your back is at a 45-degree angle and cross your arms in front of your body. Grab the handles attached to each cable. With your elbows bent slightly, pull the cables toward one another until the handles cross at the middle of your chest. Keep your hands low in front of your knees throughout the movement. Pull the cables as far as you can, then pause and lower the weights until they gently touch down. Repeat.

NOTE: Keep your back stable during the movement—don't allow your body to move up and down. Maintain steady tension on the cables throughout—don't jerk the weight up and then let it slam down on the stack. Keep your wrists firm. Your palms should be oriented toward each other as they hold the handles throughout the exercise. By keeping your body stable, you focus the effort on your pectorals. Raise and lower the weights at the same speed.

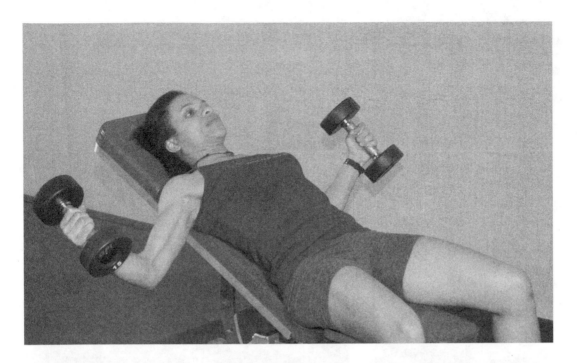

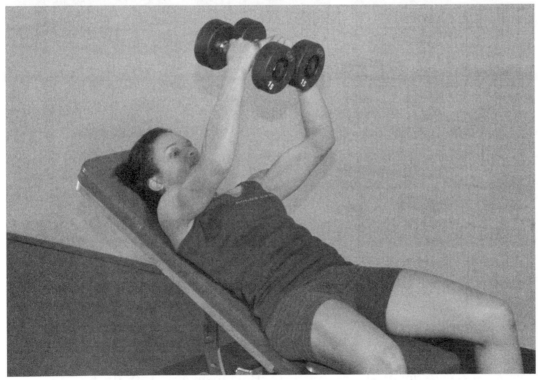

**Incline Flye**

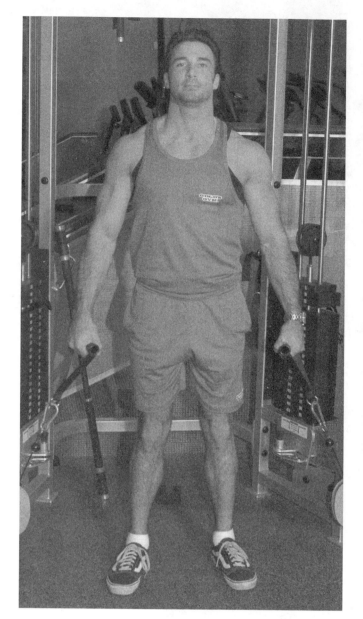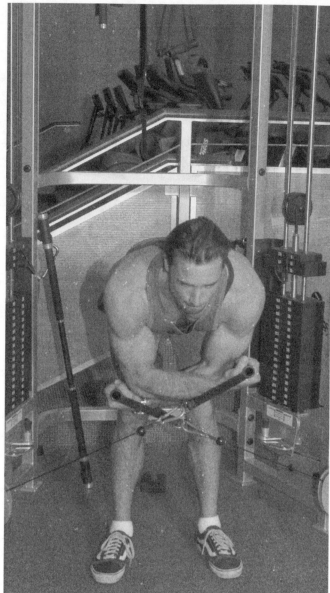

**Low-Pulley Cable Crossover**

### Lower Pecs

#### Decline Dumbbell Press

*Technique:* This is identical to the Incline Press with dumbbells, except that you lie on a decline bench, where your legs are higher than your head. By having the bench at this angle, you shift the focus to your lower pectorals. To keep your body stable during the exercise, your knees should be at the end of the bench with your lower legs hanging over the end. There should be a support bar to press your feet against for further stability and to keep you from sliding down.

Grab a dumbbell in each hand. Hold them even with the top of the bench, with your arms bent at about a 90-degree angle. Your palms should be oriented toward your feet. Press the dumbbells straight up and slightly in until your elbows lock. Let your elbows extend from your sides for better leverage. Hold, then lower the dumbbells to the starting position. Repeat.

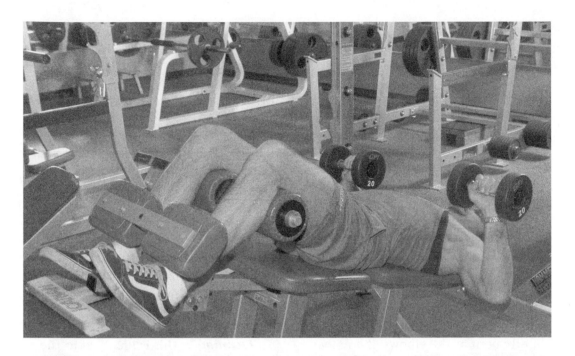

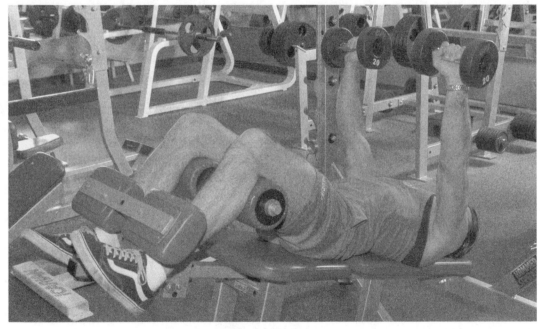

**Decline Dumbbell Press**

NOTE: Just as it takes a few sets to get used to an incline bench, it requires time to get the feel of a decline bench. A decline bench is extremely valuable, however, since it lets you develop your lower pecs far better than you can with a flat or incline bench.

As you perform this exercise, make sure that your legs are steady at the top of the bench—you don't want to slide down the bench. Use light weight in the beginning, raising and lowering the dumbbells directly over your lower chest. Don't bounce the dumbbells at the bottom of the movement; doing so would help you lift the dumbbells and thereby decrease effectiveness. You won't be able to use as much weight on a decline bench as you can on a flat bench.

### Decline Flye

*Technique:* This is a variation of the Dumbbell Flye, described in Chapter 2. Let yourself get used to the decline bench before you use heavy weight. During the exercise, keep the dumbbells in line over your lower pecs. Start with a dumbbell in each hand, with your arms bent slightly at the elbows and even with the top of the bench. Raise the dumbbells upward on a wide path until they touch over your lower pecs. Pause, then return them to your sides. Repeat.

NOTE: As with all Flye exercises, don't let the dumbbells drop too low at your sides; this could easily strain your chest muscles. Keep your arms slightly bent at the elbows; if you lock them, you make the exercise easier on your pecs.

### Bent-Forward Cable Crossover

*Technique:* This is similar to the Low-Pulley Crossover, described earlier in this chapter. The difference is that you pull the cables together and upward until they cross in front of your chest. With the Low-Pulley Crossover, you keep the cables in front of your thighs. To start this exercise, stand midway between two weight stacks, each of which has a pulley and cable attached. Place your feet slightly more than shoulder-width apart and bend your knees a little. Lean forward only slightly (not at a 45-degree angle, as with the Low-Pulley Crossover). Grab the handles attached to each cable. With your elbows bent slightly, pull the cables together and upward until the handles cross in front of your chest. Keep pulling until your arms form an X and can't go any farther. Hold, then release and slowly lower the weights to the starting position. Repeat.

NOTE: As with the Low-Pulley Crossover, keep your back stable during the movement—don't allow your body to move up and down. Maintain steady tension on the cables throughout—don't jerk the weight up and then let it slam down on the stack. Keep your wrists firm. Your palms should be oriented toward each other as they hold the handles throughout the exercise. In this exercise, feel your pectorals fully flex as your arms cross in front of your chest. Hold that flexed position before you lower the weight. Even as you tire, lower the cables steadily and at the same speed you used to raise them. If done properly, your muscles can get just as much benefit from a "negative" motion (lowering a weight) as from a "positive" motion (raising it).

### Cable Flye

*Technique:* This is identical to the Dumbbell Flye, except that you use cables instead of dumbbells. Place a flat bench midway between two weight stacks. Lie on your back and extend your arms to your sides, grabbing a handle attached to the cable with each hand and with your palms toward each other. As with the Dumbbell Flye, keep your arms bent slightly at the elbow throughout the exercise. Raise and lower the cables directly over your chest in wide arcs. Touch the handles together gently and hold for a second, then lower the weight to the starting position. Be sure to raise both cables at the same speed.

NOTE: Cables provide one benefit over dumbbells: You're able to maintain steady, constant tension throughout the exercise. With dumbbells, it's much more difficult to raise the weight than to lower it. With cables, the effort expended is about the same whether you're raising or lowering the weight. Some bodybuilders believe that cables allow you to "feel" your muscles at work more than dumbbells or barbells do. Many bodybuilders rely on free weights to build bulk and cables to shape and define their muscles, particularly before a contest.

## Inner Pecs

### *Standing Cable Crossover*

*Technique:* This exercise combines elements of the Low-Pulley Cable Crossover and the Bent-Forward Cable Crossover. The fact that there are three such similar exercises shows that slight differences in movements and angles produce significantly different results. Top bodybuilders always use multiple exercises for the same muscle to let them work the entire height and width of it. With the Standing Cable Crossover, there's a key difference from the other two crossover exercises: You use a machine that has cables attached to an overhead pulley instead of a floor-level pulley. As a result, you are pulling the cables down from above your head, instead of up from around your ankles. With this motion, you work your inner pecs more.

Here are the key differences between these cable exercises:

- **Low-Pulley Cable Crossover:** Your back is bent at a 45-degree angle. You cross the handles in front of your thighs.
- **Bent-Forward Cable Crossover:** Your back is bent forward only slightly, at about a 10- to 15-degree angle.

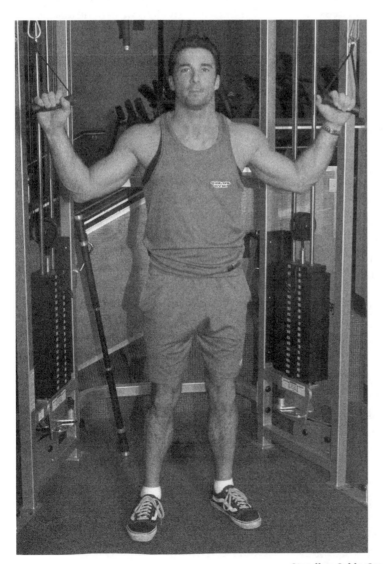
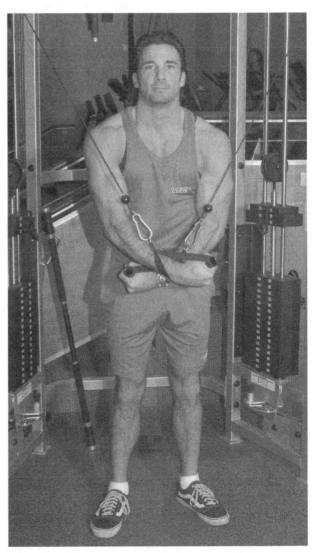

**Standing Cable Crossover**

You cross the handles in front of your chest.

- **Standing Cable Crossover:** Your back is bent at about a 30-degree angle. You cross the handles in front of your waist.

NOTE: With the Standing Cable Crossover, you need to tilt your entire body—from your feet to your head—slightly forward. This allows you to keep your balance as you raise and lower the cables from the high pulleys. In this exercise, as with the others, don't stop pulling when the handles meet in front of your body; keep pulling until your arms can't go any farther. This extra motion produces the greatest muscle benefit. For variety, alternate the way your hands cross with each rep, that is, let your right hand be in front on one rep, then your left hand on the next rep.

### Flat Bench Cable Crossover

*Technique:* This cable crossover exercise targets yet another area of your pecs. You certainly don't have to do all these different crossovers, but we're offering them for variety. People tend to find certain exercises more comfortable and effective than others. With that said, this exercise is fairly self-explanatory. Place a flat bench between two weight stacks that have floor-level pulleys. Lie on your back on the bench. Grab the handles on the cables with your palms up and straighten your arms out to the sides until your elbows almost lock. Bring the cables together over your chest until the handles barely touch. Hold, then lower the weight until your hands are even with the top of the bench.

NOTE: As a variation, you can lift the cables slightly past the point where the handles touch. By doing so, your pectoral muscles contract even more—which is the goal of all weightlifting exercises. Keep your back flat on the bench throughout the movement. Avoid the temptation to arch your back (which would make it easier to lift the weight but would reduce the effort by the pecs). As with all cable exercises, never jerk the cables up, then let them free-fall. Use a steady, gradual motion, both raising and lowering the weights. The downward motion can be just as beneficial as the upward, if done properly.

### Machine Flye

*Technique:* This exercise has an effect similar to that of the Dumbbell Flye. The difference is that you use a machine, commonly found in gyms, called a "pec deck." Sit on the seat, leaning against the seat back. (The seat height can be adjusted to fit your body.) Extend your arms to the side and bend your elbows at a 90-degree angle so that your upper arms are parallel to the floor. Place your forearms against two pads that are attached to bars, about shoulder-width apart and as high as your collarbone. Press against the pads until they meet in front of your nose. By squeezing the pads together, you raise a weight stack behind your back. Hold, then let the pads separate and return to the starting position. Repeat.

NOTE: Keep your back flat against the seat back. Lower the weights until they are 2 or 3 inches above the stack. This keeps continuous tension on your muscles—you don't rest when the weights hit the stack. In addition, it allows for a smoother start to the lifting motion. If you let the weights hit the stack, you may strain your pecs as they extend too far to the sides. Exercises on this machine won't build the pectoral mass and size that you can build with free weights. However, the pec deck can be extremely helpful in creating definition and shape in your chest. For greater control during the exercise, you can wrap your fingers around the tops of the pads.

### Narrow-Grip Bench Press

*Technique:* Bench Press is one of the most basic exercises for the chest. Normally, your hands are slightly more than shoulder-width apart on the barbell, but for this exercise, use a narrow grip, with your hands only about 12 inches apart. This shifts the effort to your inner pecs. Be aware that you won't be able to lift nearly as much weight with this grip as you can with a regular, wider grip. (With a narrow grip, your entire pecs don't assist in lifting.) Except for the different grip,

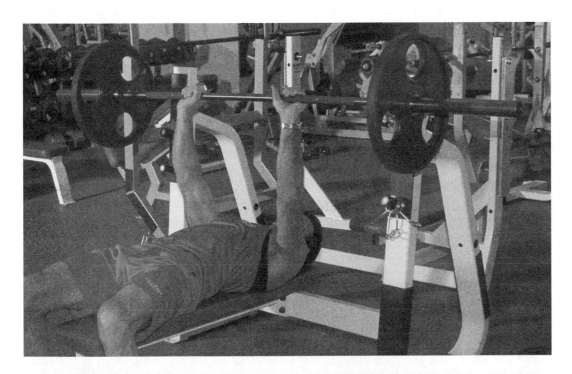

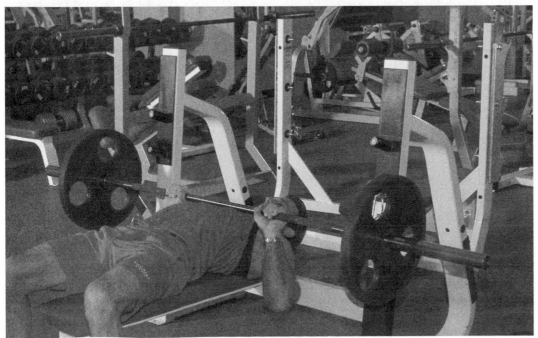

**Narrow-Grip Bench Press**

the lifting and lowering movement is the same as for regular Bench Press. Lie on your back on a flat bench, with your knees at the end of the bench and your feet on the floor. Lift the barbell off the supports overhead. Carefully bring the barbell forward until it's directly over your chest, then lower it straight down until it barely touches your chest. Push up until your arms lock. Allow your elbows to flare to the side for greater support and leverage.

NOTE: This exercise can be dangerous if done incorrectly. Because you're using a narrow grip, you don't have nearly as much control of the bar as you do with a wider grip. First and foremost, use much less weight than for regular Bench Press. Be especially careful taking the barbell off the support and bringing it forward to start the lifting movement. *Always* use a spotter for Narrow-Grip Bench Press. As you become tired, it's easy for the bar to get unbalanced and fall to one side or another, possibly injuring yourself or someone else. If you become comfortable with your hands only 12 inches apart on the bar, you can experiment with moving them closer. The closer together they are, the more your inner pecs will be worked. Be extremely careful—the narrower the grip, the more difficult it is to balance and lift the weight.

## Outer Pecs

### Flat Bench Dumbbell Press

*Technique:* This is another variation of Bench Press. Lie on a flat bench and take a dumbbell in each hand at your side, with your palms down. Extend your arms out from your body and bend your elbows at about a 90-degree angle. Gradually lift the dumbbells straight up until your elbows lock. At the top, the weights should be about 6 inches apart. Hold for a second, then lower the dumbbells to the starting position at your side. Repeat.

NOTE: Experiment with placing your feet on top of the bench, instead of on the floor. This keeps you from "cheating" with your legs—using them to help you lift the dumbbells. With your feet on the bench, your chest muscles become isolated. For more variety, you can rotate your wrists 90 degrees inward as you lift so that your palms are oriented toward each other at the top of the motion. Then you can rotate your wrists back as you lower the weight so that they're in the starting position again.

### Dips

*Technique:* This was one of the basic exercises described in Chapter 2. It doesn't use weights; instead, your body provides all the resistance. Dips are one of the best chest exercises. Almost all gyms have "dip bars"—freestanding, parallel bars that are about chest high and slightly more than shoulder-width apart.

Stand between the bars. Rise up on your toes and put your palms on top of the bars. Exhale and straighten your·arms, raising your body until your elbows lock. Your feet should be about a foot off the floor and your waist in line with the top of the bars. Hold for a second, then inhale and lower yourself gradually to the starting position, with your chest even with the bars. Bend your knees slightly to keep your feet from touching the floor. You may want to cross your ankles to keep your legs still. At the bottom, hold for a second, then exhale and push yourself back up until your elbows lock.

NOTE: Keep your torso leaning forward slightly for better balance. The more forward you can lean (while keeping your balance), the more you work your outer pecs. If you lift your ankles toward your buttocks, you'll naturally lean forward more. At first, don't lower yourself too far on the bars

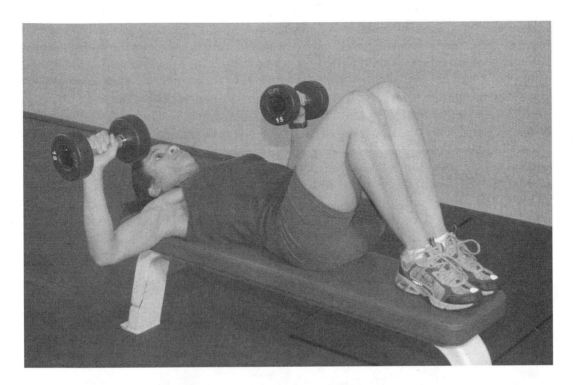

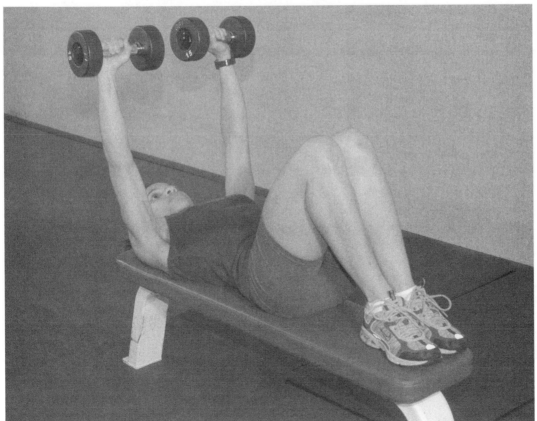

Flat Bench Dumbbell Press

or you may strain your shoulders. However, the lower you can safely go, the more your outer pecs will benefit. Some dip bars are parallel, while others have horizontal bars that taper at one end. If you use the latter, experiment with different hand positions. If you do Dips where the bars are farther apart, your outer pecs will get more work. If the bars are closer together, the effort shifts to your inner pecs. Advanced bodybuilders sometimes attach weights to their waist for greater resistance. Don't try this until you are very comfortable with regular Dips.

### Wide-Grip Incline Press

*Technique:* The Narrow-Grip Bench Press, described earlier, works the inner pecs. In this exercise, by contrast, you widen your hand position to more fully work the outer pecs. Place your hands as close to the ends of the bar as feels comfortable. Move them closer if you feel like you're straining. You won't be able to lift as much weight with a wide grip as you can with a normal, shoulder-width grip.

NOTE: Just as with the Narrow-Grip Bench Press, use light weight initially; otherwise, you can easily strain your pecs. Have a spotter nearby and wear a belt to support your back. Let your elbows flare to the sides as you lift for more control. Keep your back flat against the bench. Be sure to keep the barbell balanced as you raise and lower the weight.

# 5

# Intermediate Shoulder Exercises

"I have always emphasized deltoid training. Since my earliest days in bodybuilding, I was told that the key to a great body was to build the abdominals, calves and deltoids to the absolute maximum."

—Lee Labrada, two-time Mr. Olympia runner-up

In the previous chapter, we noted that all great bodybuilders have outstanding chests. The same can be said of the shoulders. Broad, massive shoulders are a natural complement to a thick chest.

Shoulders provide the foundation for the sharp V shape that marks a top bodybuilder—a wide upper body narrowing to a small waist. Some people are born with fairly wide shoulders, while others have to work extremely hard to achieve them.

The shoulder muscles are called deltoids, or "delts." They are large, rounded muscles at the ends of our shoulder bones. Delts lie just above the triceps—the top arm muscles—and tie into the chest muscles (pecs). Delts also join the trapezius muscles (traps) of the upper back. We include traps in our discussion of shoulder muscles because most bodybuilders exercise their delts and traps at the same time. The traps are flat, triangle-shaped muscles that start at the base of the neck in the back and extend across the shoulder blades, then down to the middle of the back. The top of the traps can be seen from the front of the body, connecting the shoulder muscles to the neck.

The deltoid is considered one muscle, but it has three distinct parts, or heads. All three heads must be fully developed for the shoulders to be considered outstanding.

The front of the deltoid is the *anterior* head, the side is the *medial* head, and the back is the *posterior* head. It's important to understand the role of each part in day-to-day functioning. The anterior head lets us raise our arms to the front of our bodies. The medial head allows us to lift our arms to the sides. The posterior head makes it possible to raise our arms behind our bodies, as a sprinter does to grab a baton in a race. All three heads work together when you extend your arms straight out from your sides and rotate them in a circle.

Some shoulder exercises work all three parts of the deltoid in varying degrees, but most exercises target one head more than the others. We'll describe exercises that work all three. Most people tend to work the front head most because it's the most visible, but you can't ignore the side and back heads if you want to be competitive in a bodybuilding contest.

Muscle proportion is critical in bodybuilding. If you develop one muscle—or a part of one muscle—more than those around it, your physique is flawed. As you gain experience, pay attention to which areas seem to be developing faster than others so that you can adjust your regimen as necessary.

Remember that weak shoulder development cannot be hidden in a contest. In virtually every pose, at least one part of the deltoid is visible. For instance, poses intended to show off chest muscles highlight the front delts. Poses for the back draw attention to the back delts. Side poses exhibit the side delts.

The entire deltoid area must be developed so that it's clearly separate from the pecs and traps. Again, definition is a key part of bodybuilding. Some people naturally have greater separation between their delts and surrounding muscles, whereas others have to work harder to achieve it.

Well-developed delts give you more than a wide look; they give you a *thick* look. Thickness, or hardness, is another essential element in bodybuilding. People often develop wide shoulders soon after they begin serious weight training, but thickness is more difficult and takes longer to achieve. Thickness separates bodybuilding champs from "wannabes."

Earlier in this book, we stressed the importance of warm-up sets to keep from straining muscles. You should use lighter weight (about half of what you would use for training) and do about twice as many reps. Warm-up sets are extremely important when working your shoulders, because your shoulders can be easily injured by lifting too much weight too soon. A strained shoulder can be slow to heal, resulting

in ongoing problems that can cause you to miss workouts.

A few minutes of warm-up sets can do wonders to prevent shoulder injuries. You can do warm-ups with any of the exercises listed below. Remember to use light weight and proper form to get the best possible warm-up.

Delts can be slow to develop. For most people, they don't grow as quickly as pecs or biceps. You need to be patient and stick with the exercises. Some bodybuilding champs worked long and hard before their delts became respectable.

The deltoid muscles are complex because they move your arms to the front, back, side, and in a circle. To work the entire deltoid area, you need to do a variety of exercises.

"I like to keep variety in my workouts so that I'm always hitting the muscles from a different angle," said Shawn Ray, two-time Mr. Olympia runner-up.

Deltoid exercises fall into two main groups: *presses* and *raises*. With presses, you lift weight directly over your head. Presses involve all three heads of the delt. With raises, you lift the weight in a wide arc to the front, side, or back of your body. Front raises strengthen the front head, side raises the medial head, and rear raises the posterior head. With raises, especially, the amount of weight you use is far less important than lifting with proper form. You want to isolate the delts as you lift without drawing on the strength of your back or legs.

"Many bodybuilders try to go too heavy when they train delts," said Steve Brisbois, a former leading bodybuilder. "The delts are actually a small muscle and don't require tons of weight to grow, but they do require high-intensity work and strict form to keep the leverage on the shoulders. I use a weight heavy enough to tax the muscle but light enough to control."

## A BRIEF HISTORY OF WOMEN'S BODYBUILDING

If men's bodybuilding has come a long way, women's bodybuilding has come light years.

The first competition for women wasn't held until the late 1970s—and contestants wore *high heels.*

In 1980, women's bodybuilding gained legitimacy when the International Federation of Bodybuilders, the sport's governing board, sanctioned the first Ms. Olympia contest—the female counterpart to the famed Mr. Olympia competition.

The first Ms. Olympia winner was Rachel McLish, whose sleek muscularity and beauty drew widespread attention to the sport. She proved that muscles and femininity can coexist.

Rachel was followed by Cory Everson, who won the Ms. Olympia title six straight times in the 1980s and became the sport's first superstar. She retired in 1990 and was quickly followed by Lenda Murray, who matched Cory's record by winning six consecutive Ms. Olympia titles in the 1990s.

Another dominant bodybuilder emerged in 1996, Kim Chizevsky. She won four straight Ms. Olympia titles and further pushed the boundaries of female muscularity. She weighed 165 pounds and had extraordinary definition.

Some people, however, criticized Kim for being too large and too muscular. Her titles intensified a debate that had been growing for years and remains unresolved. How big should women bodybuilders strive to become? Some bodybuilding fans and officials think women should get as big as they can—just like men. Others think women should strive for a leaner, more feminine appearance.

"Everyone is entitled to an opinion, but in my view, women have the same skeletal muscles as men and should be free to develop them as they wish," Arnold Schwarzenegger writes in *The New Encyclopedia of Modern Bodybuilding.*

"We live in a time in which women are becoming involved in all manner of activities and professions that were once denied to them. I am happy to see women overcoming the artificial barriers that have limited them in the past."

After Chizevsky won her fourth straight Ms. Olympia title in 1999, she retired from bodybuilding. Women with smaller muscles and a softer appearance won the next two years. Then in 2002, Lenda Murray came out of retirement and regained the Ms. Olympia crown.

Her development approached that of Chizevsky. Lenda makes no apologies for her size. "No woman in the history of the sport has displayed such astonishing symmetry and shape—wide, developed shoulders, a radically V-shaped torso, and incredibly flaring quadriceps," Lenda says on her web site. "*Muscle and Fitness* [magazine] dubbed Lenda 'the shape of things to come'."

## EXERCISES

### Front Delts

*Military Press* (illustrated on p. 27)

*Technique:* Bend your knees, lower your buttocks, and grab a barbell off the floor with an overhand grip (palms down, thumbs in). Your hands and feet should be slightly more than shoulder-width apart. Stand and carefully raise the bar to your shoulders so that it is even with your collarbone. Your palms will be under the bar for support and your elbows close against your sides. Hold the barbell for a second, then lift it straight up smoothly, keeping it close to your face, until your elbows lock. Keep the weight balanced and under control. Be careful not to lean backward or forward. At the top, hold momentarily, then lower the bar to your shoulders without bouncing it against your chest. Repeat.

NOTE: If possible, use a barbell off a shoulder-high rack for this exercise, instead of lifting one off the floor. This will help prevent lower back strain as you bring the bar to the starting position at your shoulders. Military Press can also be done while seated; this isolates your delts even more and prevents you from "cheating" with your legs.

There are specially designed benches for Military Press; they have a flat seat and a short back to help stabilize your torso as you lift. In addition, there are a variety of machines that allow you to do a Military Press lifting motion. Always wear a belt when doing any variation of this exercise, which can place a large amount of stress on your lower back. Military Press is the most basic exercise for front delt development, but it also works the side delts.

### Dumbbell Press

*Technique:* Dumbbell Press is identical to Military Press, except that it's done with dumbbells instead of a barbell. To avoid swaying, Dumbbell Press is best done while seated. Let your elbows flare to the sides to stabilize the weight as you lift. You can lift the dumbbells either one at a time or simultaneously. Some bodybuilders believe that lifting each arm separately creates a smoother, more fluid motion. Try both methods to see which you prefer.

NOTE: Wear a belt for Dumbbell Press to protect your lower back. Dumbbell Press has two advantages over presses with a barbell: You can lower the weight farther, since there's no bar in the middle to hit your chest, and you can vary the distance between your hands at the top of the movement. For instance, you can bring the dumbbells together until they touch at the top, or you can have them at shoulder width. You can also keep your palms oriented forward as you lift or rotate your wrists gradually so that your palms are oriented toward each other at the top.

### Arnold Press

*Technique:* Arnold Press is similar to Dumbbell Press, but there are several key differences. Start with the dumbbells at shoulder height with your palms oriented inward instead of for-

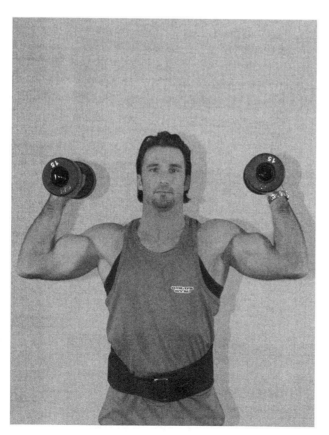
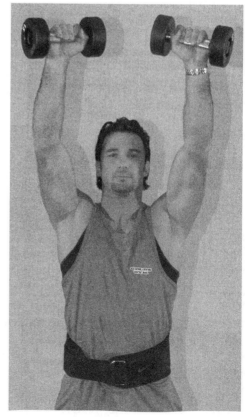

**Arnold Press**

ward. As you lift, rotate your wrists 90 degrees so that your palms are oriented forward at the top. Don't lock your elbows at the top. When you lower the dumbbells, rotate your wrists back so that your palms are oriented inward again.

NOTE: Arnold Press is named for Arnold Schwarzenegger, who popularized it. It's best done while seated for greater upper body stability. For variety, you can lower the dumbbells to your chest instead of stopping at your shoulders. This increases the range of motion and works the delts in a slightly different way.

### Front Dumbbell Raise

*Technique:* The Front Dumbbell Raise can be done while standing or seated. Hold dumbbells at your sides with your thumbs pointed toward each other. Straighten your left arm and raise it in front of your body and overhead. Pause at the top, then lower the dumbbell—under control—while

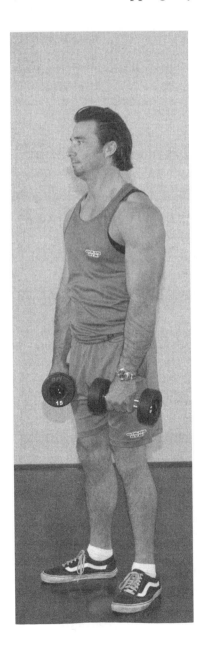
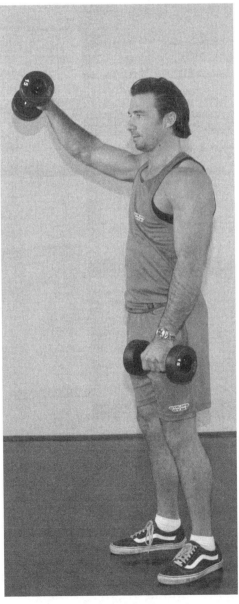
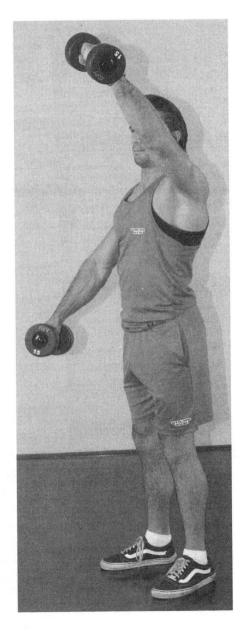

**Front Dumbbell Raise**

simultaneously raising your right arm. Both arms should be in motion at the same time, passing in front of your face. Keep your arms parallel to one another, and don't allow your torso to sway. If you do the Front Dumbbell Raise while standing, bend your knees slightly for stability.

NOTE: As you lift, you can keep your wrists in line with your forearms, or you can bend your wrists down slightly. In addition, you can rotate your wrists 90 degrees so the dumbbells are held vertically instead of horizontally. Some bodybuilders think holding them this way lessens the strain on the shoulder joint. You can also perform this lifting motion with a barbell instead of dumbbells. Use an overhand grip and keep your arms straight. Gradually raise the bar in front of your body, then to your forehead, but not all the way overhead.

### Clean and Press

*Technique:* The "clean" in Clean and Press refers to the motion of lifting the barbell off the floor and to a resting point in front of your chest. From there, you "press," or lift, the weight overhead. With each repetition, you return the barbell to the floor. That's how this exercise is different from Military Press, where you begin and end each rep with the bar at your shoulders.

Lowering yourself to the floor for each rep to "clean" the weight can be stressful on your lower back. Follow this technique to do it safely: Bend your knees fully and squat until your thighs are parallel to the floor. Lean forward slightly and grab the bar with an overhand grip and with your hands shoulder-width apart. With a smooth, steady motion, stand and lift the barbell at the same time. Bring it to the top of your chest, even with your shoulders. Pause, then lift the weight overhead under control. Pause again,

then lower the bar to your chest, bend your knees, and place the barbell back on the floor—in one continuous motion.

NOTE: Because of all the squatting and standing with Clean and Press, use extreme caution. If it continues to be awkward or painful, don't do it; there are other exercises that can produce the same results. However, some advanced bodybuilders swear by Clean and Press. They've learned to do it properly, and they say it produces thick, hard deltoids—while developing your traps, arms, and back as well. It's considered a "holistic" exercise.

## Side Delts

### *Dumbbell Lateral Raise* (illustrated on p. 68)

*Technique:* Stand with your feet shoulder-width apart and a dumbbell in each hand at your side. Bend forward slightly at the waist. Slowly raise your arms from your sides, with your elbows slightly bent. As you lift, rotate your wrists down slightly, so that the back of the dumbbell is higher than the front. Stop lifting when the dumbbells are slightly above your shoulders. Don't let your body rock. Hold the weights above your shoulders for a second, then slowly lower them to the starting position at your side. Start each new rep from a complete stop— don't swing the weight up. Keep your torso stable, maintaining a slight forward lean.

NOTE: You can do this exercise seated if you have trouble keeping your upper body stationary. If you do it properly, you should feel a slight burning sensation in the side delt. That's a good sign. Wear a belt to ease the strain on your lower back. For variety, you can bring the dumbbells down toward the front of your body instead of to the side. In addition, you can bend your elbows at a 90-degree angle instead of keeping your arms straight.

### Cable Lateral Raise

*Technique:* The Cable Lateral Raise is very similar to the Dumbbell Lateral Raise, except that you use a machine with a cable. Cables provide the advantage of continuous, steady tension as you raise and lower the weight. Unlike the Dumbbell Lateral Raise, you work one arm at a time with the Cable Lateral Raise. Stand with the right side of your body about a foot from the weight stack. Grab the handle with your left hand, so that your left arm crosses in front of your chest.

*Note:* The models are not wearing belts in the photographs in this chapter because they are lifting light weight for demonstration purposes.

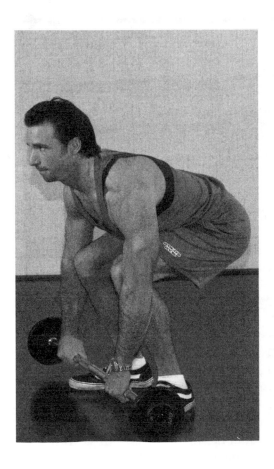

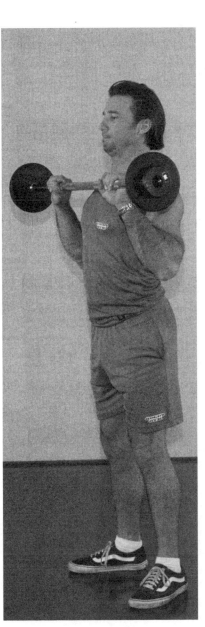

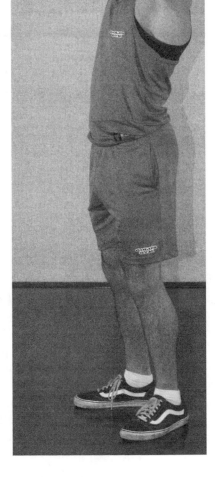

**Clean and Press**

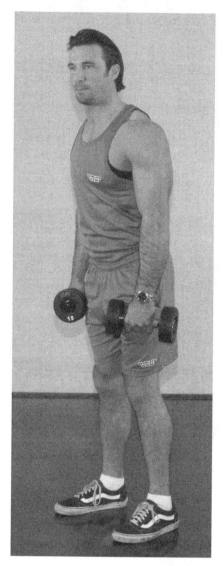
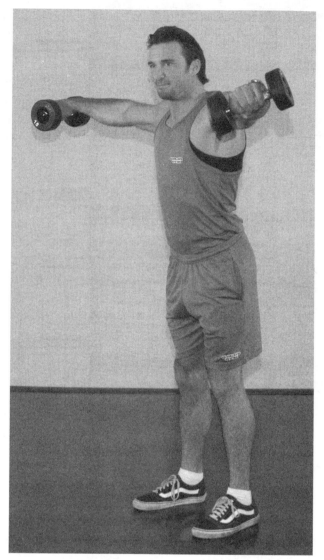

**Dumbbell Lateral Raise**

Bend your right arm and place your right hand on your hip for stability. With your left elbow bent, pull the cable out and up until your left hand is higher than your shoulder. As you lift, twist the front of your wrist down slightly (as if pouring water from a pitcher). When you finish the reps, stand with the left side of your body about a foot from the weight stack. Lift the cable with your right hand in the same manner as with your left.

NOTE: Don't let your body sway while lifting. Use only your deltoid. As you lower the weight, let the handle drop slightly below the middle of your torso. Let the weights touch down only

slightly before lifting again. You can also lift while sitting. For more variety, you can step forward a few inches and lift the cable *behind* your body instead of in front.

### Lying Side Lateral

*Technique:* The Lying Side Lateral combines elements of the Dumbbell Lateral Raise and the Cable Lateral Raise. Lie on a bench (either flat or incline) on your right side. Hold a dumbbell in your left hand near or slightly below your hip. Your elbow should be slightly bent. Lower the dumbbell in front of your body until it's about 6 inches from the floor.

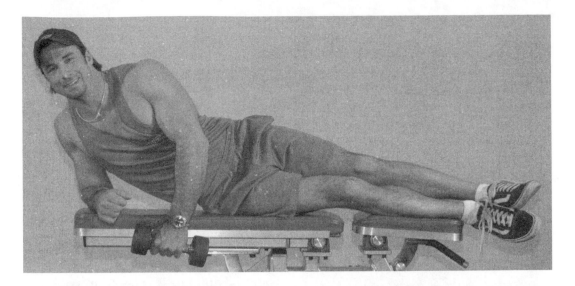

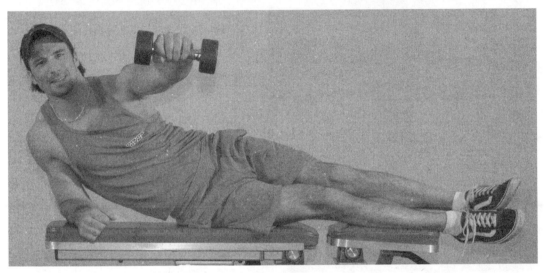

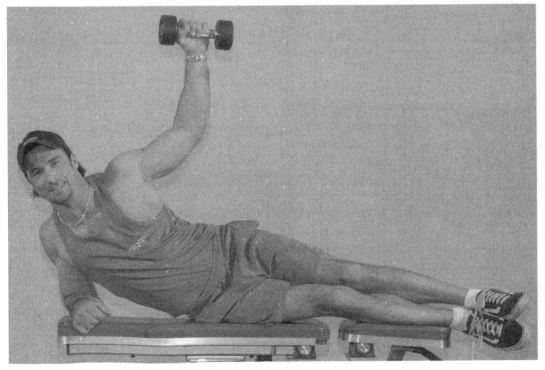

**Lying Side Lateral**

Pause, then lift your arm straight up until it's directly overhead. The front of the dumbbell should point down slightly or be parallel to the floor. When you finish the reps, turn and lie on your right side. Repeat the exercise with your right hand.

NOTE: Use light weight so that you can perform the motion properly. By lying on a bench instead of the floor, you have a greater range of motion.

### Prone Dumbbell Lateral Raise

*Technique:* Lie face down on an incline bench with your head at the top. Grab a dumbbell in each hand and let your arms hang loosely down with your palms oriented toward each another. Bend your elbows slightly and raise the dumbbells away from your sides and upward in a wide arc. Stop when the weights are just above your shoulders. Lift gradually and under control. As you near the top, turn the front of the dumbbells down slightly to focus effort on the side delt. At the top, hold the dumbbell for a moment, then lower it along the same path until it's about 2 inches below the bench.

## Rear Delts

### Bent-Over Dumbbell Lateral Raise

*Technique:* Do this exercise while seated. It's identical to the Dumbbell Lateral Raise, described above, except that you bend forward at the waist at about a 45-degree angle to work the back part of the delt.

NOTE: Keep in mind the following points:

1. Sit with your feet close together and your knees almost touching.
2. Start with the dumbbells behind your calves and return them there, until they almost touch.
3. Don't raise your body as you lift—this would reduce the benefit to your delts.
4. Raise the dumbbells just above head high.
5. Keep the dumbbells in line with your shoulders throughout the movement, with your palms oriented toward each other. Don't let the dumbbells drift behind your shoulders.

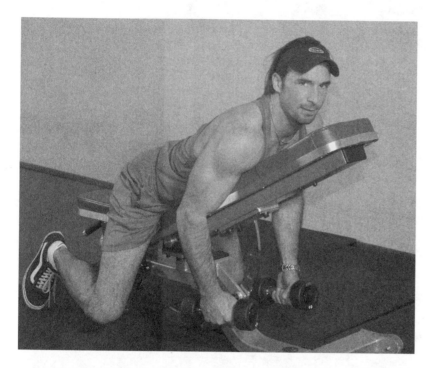

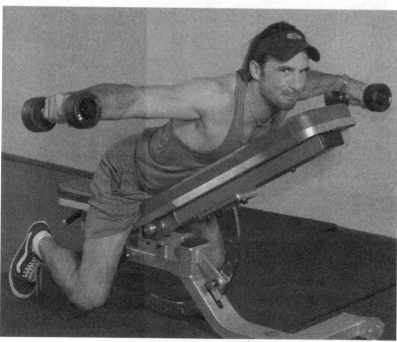

**Prone Dumbbell Lateral Raise**

6. At the top of the movement, pause, then lower the dumbbells under control.

### Bent-Over Cable Lateral Raise

*Technique:* This exercise is similar to the Cable Lateral Raise. The key differences are that with the Bent-Over Cable Lateral Raise, you use two cables instead of one and you lift with both arms at the same time.

Stand midway between two weight stacks, with your feet shoulder-width apart. Cross your arms in front of your body in an X and grab the handles. Your left hand will hold the handle on your right side, and your right hand will hold the handle on your left side. Bend from the waist until your back is almost parallel to the floor. Pull your arms simultaneously out and up in a wide, smooth motion until they are above your head. Pause, then let the weights lower and your hands cross in front of your body.

NOTE: You should feel continuous, steady tension on your rear delts throughout this exercise. Don't raise your torso; keep it almost parallel to the floor—this keeps the effort on the rear delt.

### Bent-Over Row (illustrated on p. 72)

*Technique:* Grab a barbell with an overhand grip and your hands 8 to 10 inches apart. Stand with your feet slightly more than shoulder-width apart. Bend your torso forward at a 45-degree angle. Keeping your legs and upper body stationary, lift the barbell straight up until it touches the top of your abs. Hold momentarily, then lower it under control, stopping in front of your shins.

NOTE: A similar exercise, the Upright Row, is a classic for lat and trap development. By bending your torso forward, you shift the effort to your rear delts. Be sure to lift the barbell only as high as your upper abs—not all the way

to your chest. This also helps the exercise benefit your delts instead of your lats and traps. Keep your head up and your eyes looking forward throughout the movement to reduce strain on your

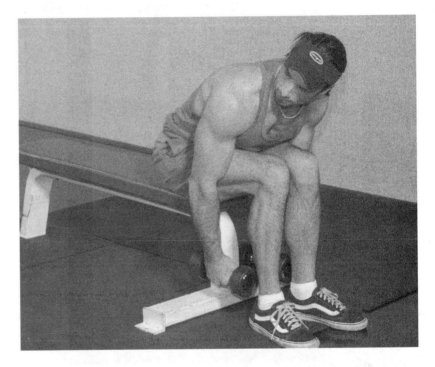

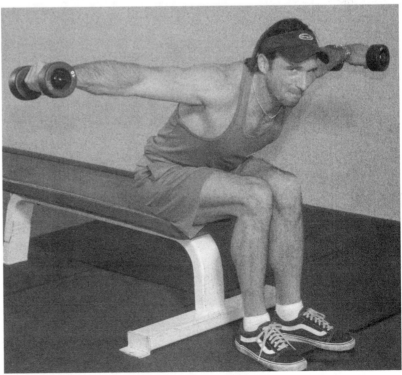

**Bent-Over Dumbbell Lateral Raise**

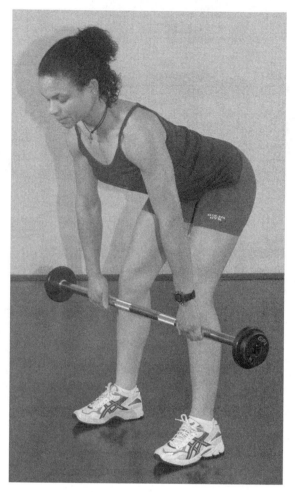
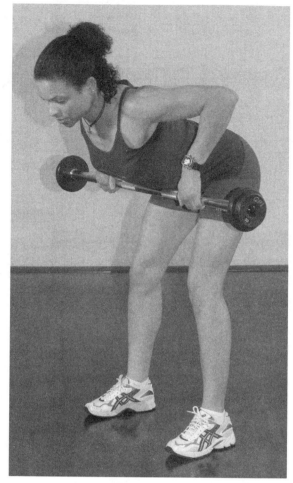

**Bent-Over Row**

neck. Wear a belt to protect your lower back.

### Prone Dumbbell Lateral Raise

*Technique:* Sit at the end of a flat bench. Place your feet close together on the floor. Lean over until your torso rests against your thighs. Holding a dumbbell in each hand, let your arms hang straight down with your palms oriented toward each other. Bend your elbows slightly, then lift the dumbbells up and out, keeping them in line with your shoulders. Stop when the weights reach head high. Pause, then lower the dumbbells gradually to the starting position.

NOTE: Keep your torso stationary during the movement. For variety, you can raise the dumbbells a little

to the front of your shoulders, instead of in line with them.

## Traps

### Upright Row

*Technique:* Grab a barbell with an overhand grip and your hands 8 to 10 inches apart. Stand with your feet slightly more than shoulder-width apart and the barbell resting against the front of your body. Keep your legs stationary and your back straight. Lift the barbell straight up—keeping it close to your torso—until it almost touches your chin. Hold momentarily, then lower it under control to a position just below your waist.

NOTE: Keep your head up and your eyes looking forward throughout the exercise. This isolates your traps instead

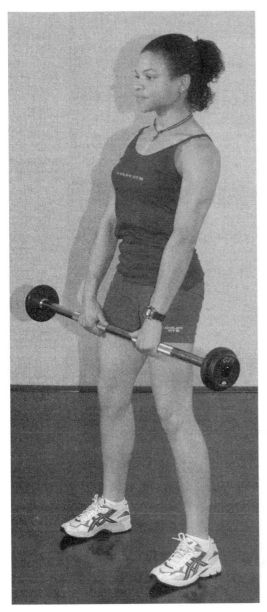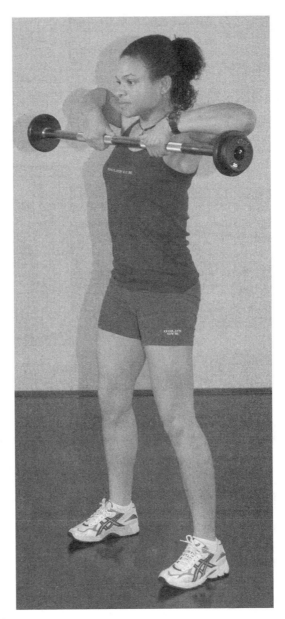

**Upright Row**

of allowing your entire torso to lift the weight. Wear a belt to stabilize your lower back.

### Shrugs (illustrated on p. 74)

*Technique:* Grab a barbell with an overhand grip and your hands shoulder-width apart. Let the bar rest against your thighs. Lift or "shrug" your shoulders as high as you can, as if they are going to touch your ears. Keep your lower body steady and arms bent slightly at the elbows. Don't sway.

When your shoulders are at the highest point, pause momentarily, then gradually lower your shoulders and the bar to the starting position.

NOTE: This is a very short movement. The bar rises only 4 to 6 inches as you shrug your shoulders. The distance is not important—proper form is. Your traps can get a great workout with very little movement. As you lift, dip your chin toward your chest slightly. This helps stabilize your torso and focuses the effort on the traps

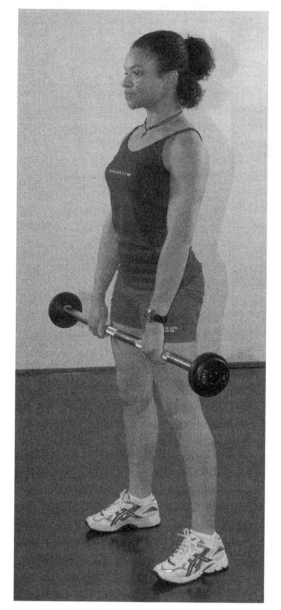 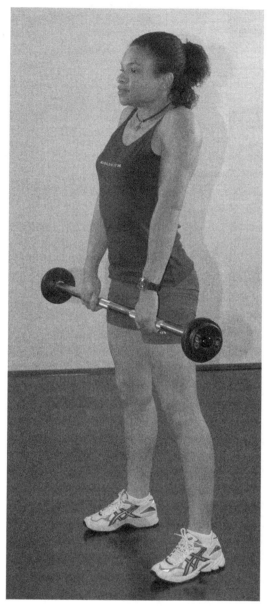

**Shrugs**

instead of the chest or delts. You can try a wider or narrower grip to work different areas of the traps. Wear a belt to protect your lower back. Shrugs can also be done with dumbbells. However, hold them at your sides, not in front. Let your arms hang straight down throughout the motion. Some people find this exercise more comfortable and effective with dumbbells because they allow you to have a longer range of motion.

### Lying Incline Lateral

*Technique:* Lie face down on an incline bench with your head at the top. Hold a dumbbell in each hand with your palms oriented toward each other. Let your arms hang down loosely. Bend your elbows slightly, then raise your arms out and up in a wide arc until they are slightly above and in front of your shoulders. They should be in line with your ears. At the top, twist the front of the dumbbells down

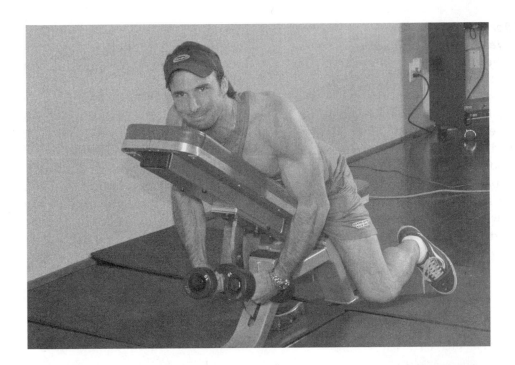

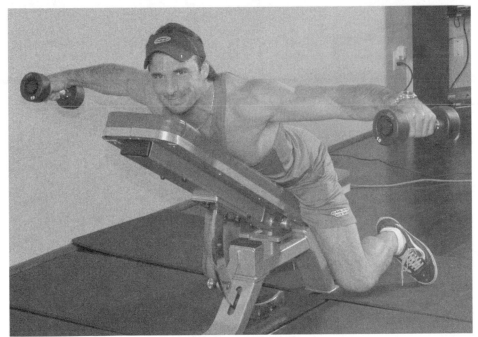

**Lying Incline Lateral**

slightly to more fully work the traps. Hold for a second, then gradually lower the dumbbells to the starting position.

NOTE: In the first part of this exercise, your delts will do most of the work. As your arms approach the topmost position, your traps come into play. At the very highest point, you should feel your traps fully contract. Be sure to keep the dumbbells in line with your ears, not back a few inches (in line with your shoulder joints). That small difference causes your traps to work more than your delts.

### T-Bar Row

*Technique:* This exercise is similar to the Upright Row, except that you don't use a barbell. Instead, you use a piece of equipment that has a long metal bar (longer than a barbell), with one end hinged at the floor. Place weights on the free end. Step onto a wooden box or platform and straddle the bar. Bend your knees slightly, lean over and grab a short bar that forms a T with the long bar. Pull the weights toward your chest. Keep your back bent at a 45-degree angle. Lift until the weights touch your chest. Pause, then lower the weights, straightening your arms.

NOTE: Keep your head up and your eyes looking forward during the T-Bar Row to ease the strain on your neck. Pull your shoulders back slightly as you lift. Don't let your body sway. If you can't remain stationary, you're using too much weight; remove some weight until you can lift with proper form.

# 6

# Intermediate Back and Neck Exercises

"My back is a weapon I use to destroy my opponents."
—Franco Columbo, two-time Mr. Olympia

"Thick" and "wide"—those are the two words most commonly used to describe outstanding back development. An awe-inspiring back can be the final piece of the puzzle needed to achieve bodybuilding success. Too often, young bodybuilders—and even seasoned veterans—overlook the back in their workouts.

The reason is simple. Bodybuilding judges, as well as others, tend to notice a person's chest and shoulders first. It takes a trained eye to appreciate the less-obvious, less-dramatic group of muscles that make up the back. Yet a broad back is the key to the extreme V shape that bodybuilders need—an expansive upper torso that tapers to a narrow waist. Well-developed "lats"—the muscles that flare out from the sides of the torso—are clearly visible from the front and play a key role in a number of mandatory poses in competition.

Don't spend so much effort on the "showy" muscles—the chest, shoulders, biceps, and legs—that you don't have enough time to properly train the back.

Some people become discouraged because back muscles often develop more slowly than other muscles, which can seem to pop out quickly with serious training. It may take years of concentrated training to build a championship-caliber back. As a beginning bodybuilder, you should make the commitment to train the back as seriously as any other part of your body. Don't worry if you fail to see immediate results. If you're doing the correct exercises with proper form, you'll make progress—even though the payoff may be farther down the road.

By making your back a priority early on, you'll avoid a problem that some advanced bodybuilders face. They reach the upper levels of the sport only to find that their underdeveloped backs are keeping them from becoming winners.

"The most common problem of today's competition bodybuilders is incomplete back development," Arnold Schwarzenegger says. "Back training is more subtle and more difficult than most people realize."

## MUSCLES OF THE BACK

Before you can hope to sculpt a massive, "ripped" back, you have to understand the muscles that comprise it. To simply say "back muscles" is too general and too oversimplified to be useful. Unless you understand each muscle and its function, you can't target it with specific exercises.

### Latissimus Dorsi

Commonly called the "lats," these are the triangle-shaped muscles that extend from below the armpits to the lower back on both sides. They are the largest muscles of the back and the only ones that can be clearly seen in a frontal view. Often the lats aren't prominent when bodybuilders are in a relaxed position. When flexed, however, the lats spread out like wings under the arms. People who don't train with weights usually have little lat development, so when you see someone with prominent lats, you know you're looking at a bodybuilder.

Strong lat muscles aren't just for show. They let you pull your arms backward, and they allow you to lift and carry heavy weight without straining your lower back. To develop great lats, you need to do exercises with a pull-down movement, such as Chin-Ups. Another exercise is the Cable Pull-down—you grab a long bar overhead and press it down toward the floor, raising a weight stack.

You can work different areas of the lats by varying the grip and the lifting motion when doing the exercises. For instance, if you do the Cable Pull-down with the bar in front of your head, you get one result. If you do it by pulling the bar *behind* your head, you get another.

Over the years, advances in training methods have contributed to better and better back development. Look at today's bodybuilding superstars—their backs are so broad that they dwarf the backs of top competitors from just a few decades ago.

Lats have distinct upper and lower parts. The lower lats extend from the middle of the back almost to the waist. To develop them, you'll do exercises with a narrow grip. Chin-Ups and Cable Pulldowns are excellent when you bring your hands close together. These same exercises, and many more, build the upper lats by using a much wider grip.

### Upper Back

The muscles of the upper, center part of the back are called the trapezius muscles, or "traps." They are flat and triangular, starting at the base of the neck and extending horizontally across the shoulder blades and vertically down to the middle of the spine. Traps allow you to pull your shoulders up and back. Although the traps are technically muscles of the back, bodybuilders train them with their shoulder muscles. We included several trap exercises, such as Shrugs and Upright Rows, in the previous chapter. Review them if necessary.

Well-developed traps provide a clear center line to your back that highlights broad lats on either side. Your traps must be well-defined and distinctly separate from your lats.

### Middle Back

Of all the back muscles, those of the middle back may be the most ignored. You can easily spot wing-like lats and tall traps, but the middle back muscles often get lost in the mix. They are subtle, yet they must become thick and prominent to complete your back development. Someone who does not have a good middle back will pale in comparison to someone who does, although you may not immediately be able to identify why. Judges, however, are trained to spot every flaw, and their eyes quickly go to the middle back when sizing up competitors.

To develop the muscles of the middle back, you need to do exercises that involve a long range of motion. Extreme pulling and stretching movements call the middle back muscles into action. A good example is the Cable Row. You sit on the floor (or on a seat) facing a weight stack and pull two cables toward your chest. The exercise requires you to fully straighten and extend your arms as you return the weight, then pull your arms as far back as possible to lift the weight.

### Lower Back

An outstanding lower back is marked by two thick vertical columns of muscles on either side of the lower spine; these are called spinal erectors. They start about 4 inches above your waist and extend below your waistline. Spinal erectors help you to arch your spine to perform many day-to-day functions. They stabilize your lower torso and protect your spine from injury. They don't flex in dramatic fashion, like biceps or lats. Although they tend to keep their shape whether you're relaxing or working out, they must be prominent if you are to have a fully developed back.

Spinal erectors can easily become strained, or even seriously injured, by improper lifting or by too much work. Yet they are critical in helping to avoid lower back problems, which are common to many people. The more you can develop these muscles, the less likely you are to develop these back problems.

When you first begin to work your lower back, warm up thoroughly and proceed carefully. You don't need a great deal of weight to build your spinal erectors, given their small size. Proper form is much more important. Bring

these muscles along slowly as you sculpt your entire physique, but make sure that you don't ignore them. They can become a weak link in your back development if you don't target them in training.

As Schwarzenegger says, "If you don't properly appreciate the complexity of the back and how many different movements it takes to get full back development, you will end up with serious weak points in this part of your physique."

## BACK EXERCISES

### Lats

#### Lat Pulldown

*Technique:* This exercise is done on a machine found in almost every gym. A long horizontal overhead bar is attached to a cable that ties into a stack of weights. Crouch down on your knees under the bar, or sit on a seat if one is provided. Raise your arms overhead and grab the bar with a wide overhand grip—about 2 to 3 inches from the ends. Angle your torso back slightly and pull the bar down smoothly in front of your face until it touches the top of your chest. Hold for a second, then gradually let the bar rise back to its starting position.

NOTE: Keep your torso steady. Don't let your torso sway backward—doing so takes effort off the lats and shifts it to the upper back. When your torso is steady, the lats do all the pulling. If you have trouble remaining stationary, have a spotter gently place his or her hands on your shoulders. Keep steady tension on the weights as you return them to the starting position. Don't let go of the bar and let the weights slam down. You should keep the same tension on the cable as you lift and then lower the weights. Some lat machines have a short, inverted

V–shaped handle instead of a long bar. To use this type of handle, grasp both sides of the V and perform the exercise as with the straight bar. Because you're using a much narrower grip, your lower lats will get more of a workout. If your gym doesn't have a V handle, you can accomplish the same result by bringing your hands closer together on a straight bar. You can also experiment with an underhand grip (palms up, thumbs out) on a straight bar.

### Machine Pullover

*Technique:* This exercise is also performed on a machine that's found in most gyms. You begin by sitting on a seat that has a back. Above your head is a large U-shaped bar, with the open part of the U facing out. Place your elbows on the two pads at the open end. Press down firmly on the pads with your upper arms, lowering the U-shaped bar toward your chest. Stop when it touches your abs.

NOTE: The bar moves in a semicircular motion from start to finish. While pressing down on the bar, you can wrap your fingers around the top of the bar for a firmer hold. Keep your back firmly against the back of the seat.

If a pullover machine is not available in your gym, you can do essentially the same exercise with a barbell. Start by lying on your back on a flat bench, with your head slightly off one end. Grab a barbell and hold it behind your head, off the floor. Bend your arms at a 90-degree angle and keep them close to your sides. Smoothly lift the barbell over your head and toward your chest, stopping when it touches your chest. You may want a spotter to press down gently on your thighs so your body doesn't rise off the bench. A word of caution: If you're using a high bench, don't try to reach behind and grab a barbell off the floor. You can strain your lats doing so. Instead, have someone hand you the barbell.

### One-Arm Cable Row

*Technique:* Use a machine with a floor-level pulley. Either sitting or standing, grab the handle with your right hand (thumb up). Pull the cable toward your right side, stopping when the handle touches your ribs. Your elbow should be well behind your torso. If you do this exercise while standing, place your feet even or with your left foot well in front of your right for greater balance as you pull the cable. If you do this exercise while sitting, rest your left forearm on your left knee for more stability. When you've finished the reps, change sides and pull with your left hand.

NOTE: This exercise is particularly effective in developing your upper lats. Because of the long range of motion from start to finish, you get more benefit than with most other exercises. For variety, you can gradually twist the handle toward your torso as you lift, so that your thumb is at your side when you finish.

### Chin-Ups (illustrated on p. 82)

*Technique:* Like Dips, this versatile exercise doesn't use weights; your body provides all the resistance. Many of us are familiar with this exercise from school gym class. You stand under a horizontal bar that's anywhere from a few inches to a foot or more above your head.

Raise your arms overhead and grab the bar with a wide overhand grip (palms down, thumbs in). Your hands should be slightly more than shoulder-width apart. Make sure you have a firm grip, then pull your body up until your upper chest touches the bar and your chin is above it. As you do so, bend your knees and cross your ankles to keep your lower body steady. Keep your elbows behind your torso as you lift. At the topmost position, hold for a second, then lower yourself to the starting position.

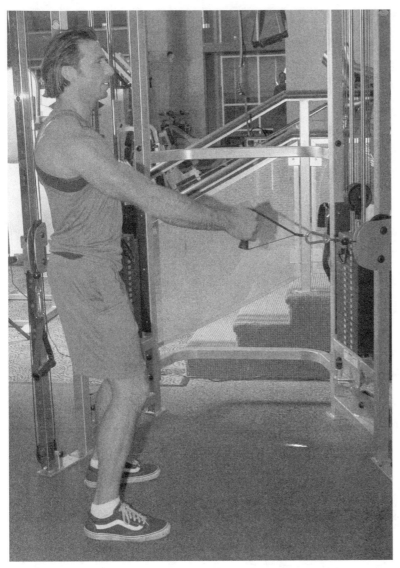
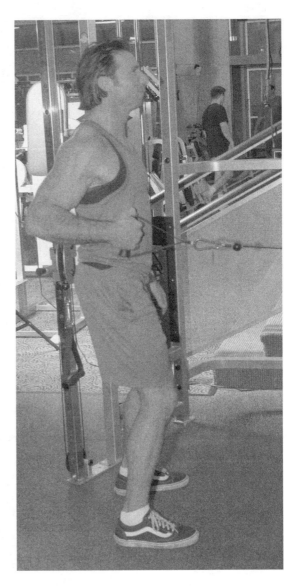

**One-Arm Cable Row**

NOTE: Chin-Ups are very difficult for some people, particularly those who are heavy. In fact, you may not be able to do a single chin-up at first. If so, skip this exercise until you build your strength with other exercises, and then try it again. If you can do Chin-Ups, try to straighten your arms almost completely as you lower yourself. This gives your lats a good stretch. However, keep your lats flexed as you hang so that your shoulder joints don't bear all the weight of your body.

For variety, you can adjust your grip so that it is wider or narrower.

The wider the grip, the more you work your upper lats. If you're especially strong, you can put your head in front of the bar (instead of behind) and lift until the back of your neck touches the bar (instead of your chin touching the bar). Some advanced bodybuilders attach weights to their waist to increase the resistance.

A word of caution: If you're using a bar that's much higher than your head, be careful as you reach for it to start the exercise—either stand on a stool or have someone assist you as you jump up to grab the bar.

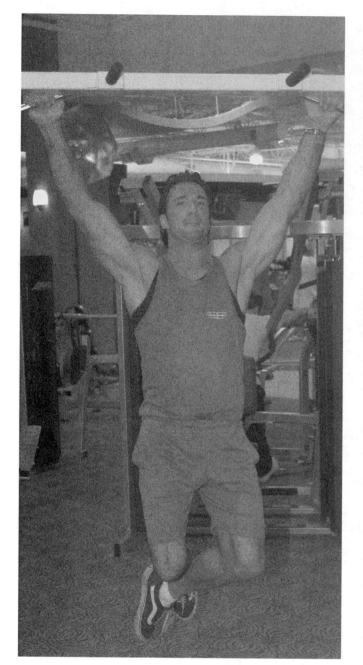
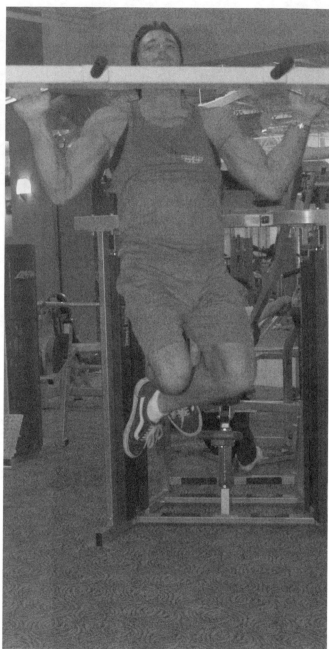

**Chin-Ups**

### Middle Back

#### *Seated Cable Row*

*Technique:* The Seated Cable Row is similar to the One-Arm Cable Row described above for lats. The main differences are that you pull with two hands simultaneously and that you are seated instead of standing. Use a machine with a floor-level pulley. Sitting on or just off the floor, bend your knees slightly and place your feet against a horizontal bar for support. Grab the V-shaped handle, holding it with your thumbs up. Lean back slightly, then pull the cable toward your ribs. Arch your back slightly and draw your shoulder blades together. Keep your arms close to your sides. Stop when the handles touch your abs; at this point your elbows should be well

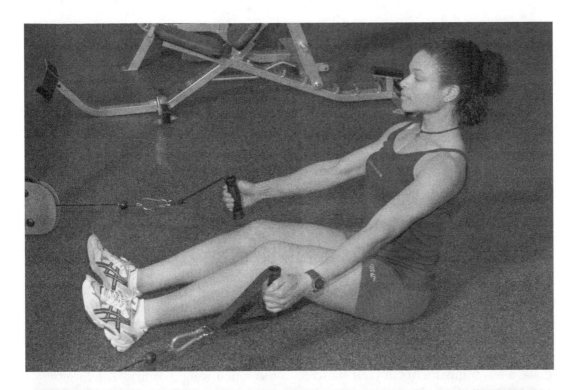

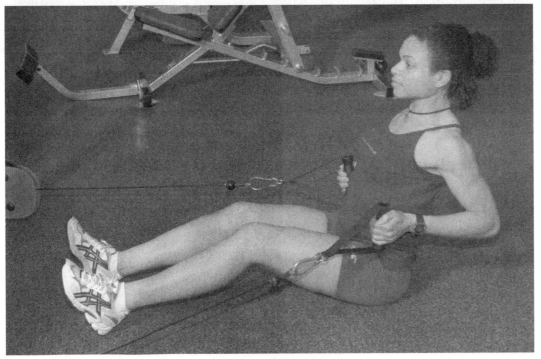

**Seated Cable Row**

behind your torso. Hold, then gradually return the weights to the starting position.

Some machines have two cables and two handles. With others, a single cable splits into two short cables that are connected to one handle. With either type, the lifting motion is the same.

NOTE: This exercise has a shorter range of motion than the One-Arm

Cable Row. Therefore, it works the middle back more than the lats, although the lats do get some benefit. As you pull the cables, lean back slightly, but then straighten your torso at the end. This lets your back muscles get more work, rather than your lats. When you lower the weight, be sure to extend your arms fully and lean forward to completely stretch your lats. For variety, you can gradually twist the handle toward your body as you lift so that your thumb is at your side as you finish.

### T-Bar Row

*Technique:* We recommended this exercise for trap development in Chapter 5, but it's also good for strengthening the middle back if you make a few adjustments in your stance and lifting motion. As a reminder, the T-Bar Row is similar to the Upright Row except that you don't use a barbell. Instead, you use a machine that has a long metal bar with one end hinged at the floor. On the other end of the bar, you load weights. You step onto a wooden box or platform, straddling the bar. With your knees bent only slightly, lean over and grab the crossbar that serves as a handle. For middle back development, tilt your torso at about a 60-degree angle (in contrast to the 45-degree angle when working the traps). Place your weight mainly on your heels. Gradually pull the bar toward you and squeeze your shoulder blades together. Lift until the weight touches your lower chest. (For trap work, you pull the bar to your mid-chest.)

NOTE: Keep your back steady with your weight toward your heels as you lift. If your weight moves toward the front of your feet, the focus shifts to your traps. Lower the weight if you have trouble remaining stationary as you lift.

### Bent-Over Row

*Technique:* The Bent-Over Row can work well to develop your rear deltoids, but it's also excellent to strengthen your middle back. Grab a barbell with an overhand grip and with your hands near the ends of the bar. Lean over from the waist so that your torso is almost parallel to the floor. Bend your knees slightly for stability. The barbell is in front of your shins. Lift it straight up until it touches the top of your abs. Hold for a moment, then lower it under control to your shins. Repeat.

NOTE: It's important to keep your head up and your eyes looking forward as you lift; this reduces strain on your neck. Keep your buttocks and thighs steady. Always wear a belt to protect your lower back, and don't try to lift too much weight at first. For variety, you can do the Bent-Over Row with a dumbbell instead of a barbell. As with all dumbbell exercises, you'll get a longer range of motion. To use a dumbbell, lean over in the same way, but place your right knee and right palm on a flat bench. This will keep your body steady as you lift a dumbbell with your left arm. Raise it from the top of the bench toward your armpit in a sawing motion. When you've finished your reps, reverse and lift with your right arm, placing your left knee and palm on the bench.

### Lower Back

**Deadlift** (illustrated on p. 86)

*Technique:* Grab a barbell on the floor with an overhand grip (palms down, thumbs in) or a "mixed grip" (one palm down, the other up). Some people find that a mixed grip allows them to lift more weight. Either way, the next step is to crouch down, bending your knees until your thighs are almost parallel to the floor. Your back should be at about a 45-degree angle. Keep your head up and your

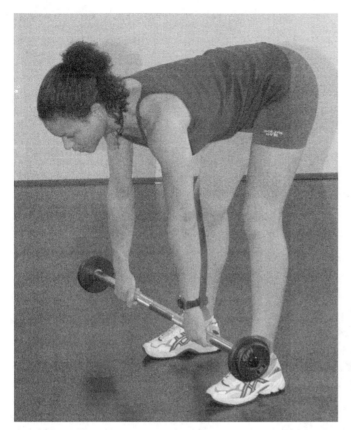 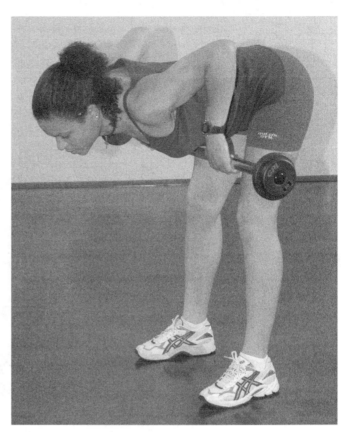

**Bent-Over Row**

*Note:* The models are not wearing belts in the photographs in this chapter because they are lifting light weight for demonstration purposes.

eyes looking forward. Begin lifting the barbell, driving up with your legs, and gradually straightening your back and knees. Keep your arms straight. As you finish lifting, pull your shoulders back and thrust your chest forward to stand fully erect. The barbell will rest against your thighs. Pause, then carefully bend your knees, lean forward from the waist, and set the barbell on the floor. With each repetition, you place the barbell on the floor and start the entire lifting motion again.

NOTE: The Deadlift is a tried-and-true exercise that involves not only your lower back but also your upper back, traps, buttocks, and legs. It's been a staple of bodybuilding champs for generations. However, if you don't use proper form, it's easy to injure your back. Always wear a weightlifting belt. Never drop your head and look down as you lift. This makes your torso lean forward too much and places stress on your lower back. Instead, keep your back at a 45-degree angle, your head up, and your eyes looking forward. Never jerk the barbell off the floor or let it drop to the floor as you finish. Don't use heavy weight until you become comfortable with the lifting motion. Pay special attention to your knees as you do the Deadlift. Some people find that this exercise hurts their knees. If it hurts your knees, don't do it. However, you might first try wrapping your knees with an elastic bandage for the exercise. Many bodybuilders do this to support their knees and avoid problems with them.

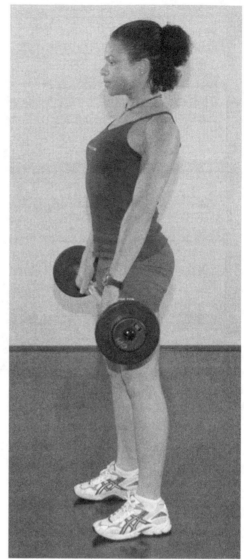

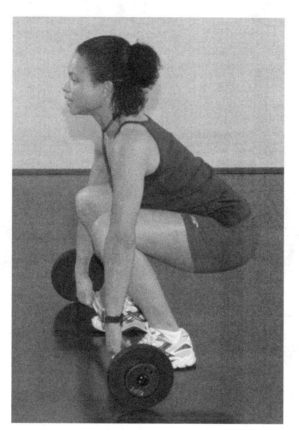

**Deadlift**

### *Good Morning*

*Technique:* This oddly named exercise is a key part of many bodybuilders' routine. (The term comes from the "rising up" motion—as if you're getting out of bed.)

Rest a barbell across the back of your shoulders behind your head, as you would with Squats. It's best to take a barbell off a rack instead of lifting it off the floor. Place your feet at shoulder width and lock your knees. Make sure you have a firm grip on the bar, then bend forward from the waist until your torso is parallel to the floor. Keep your knees locked and don't let the barbell roll onto your neck. Once you've bent over, pause, then straighten up until you are standing erect again. Keep your head up and your eyes looking forward throughout.

NOTE: Start with very light weight to get the feel of this exercise. You never want to bend over and find that you're holding too much weight, which can cause you to lose your balance and fall. Use a spotter for safety.

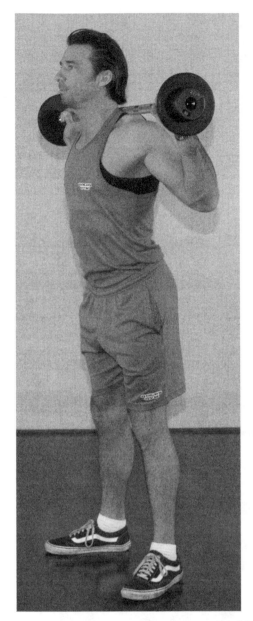
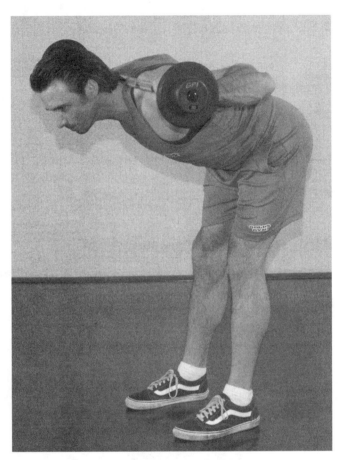

**Good Morning**

### Hyperextension (illustrated on p. 88)

**Technique:** Like Dips and Chin-Ups, this exercise uses only your body weight for resistance. The equipment specially designed for this exercise has a small pad at its top and a horizontal bar at its foot. Position yourself so that the fronts of your thighs are against the pad and your ankles are under the bar (for stability); your torso will be unsupported. Cross your arms over your chest, then bend your torso down until your head almost touches the floor. Feel your lower back muscles work. Pause, then gradually raise your torso until it's in a straight line with your legs.

NOTE: Make sure your feet and ankles are firmly under the support bar. Otherwise, you'll be unsteady and you might even fall as you perform this exercise. Lower your torso slowly

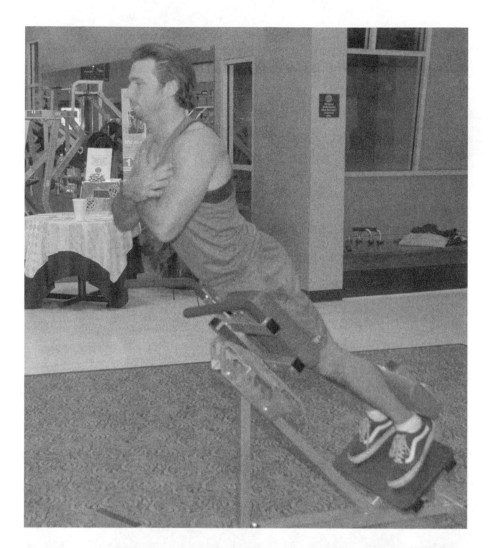

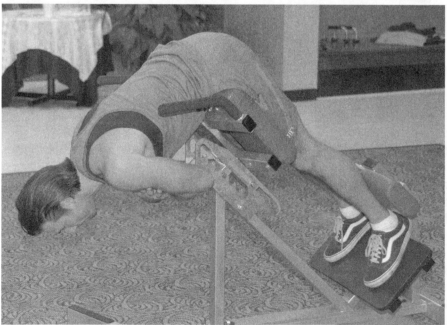

**Hyperextension**

and under control—don't let it drop quickly. Likewise, don't jerk your torso as you raise it back up. Keep your head up and your eyes looking forward. When you reach the top, don't lift your torso higher than the plane of your legs—that places too much stress on your spine. As an alternative, you can clasp your hands behind your head (instead of crossing your arms over your chest) to keep your upper body steady.

## MUSCLES OF THE NECK

Neck muscles, like those of the lower back, are often ignored. Some bodybuilders become so focused on developing the more prominent muscles that they fail to work on subtle muscles, such as those of the neck, that would complete their development. Some beginners aren't even aware that the neck can be made larger.

A powerful neck is important because it enhances the appearance of broad shoulders and a thick chest. If two people with identical shoulder and chest development stand side by side, the one with the larger neck will seem much bigger.

Football players often have large necks, and you, too, can achieve a similar look. Your neck should be only an inch or two smaller in circumference than your biceps. If your biceps are 18 inches in circumference, your neck should measure about 17 inches. If your neck measures only 15 inches, which is normal for many people, your physique will look unbalanced and out of proportion.

Fortunately, neck muscles are some of the easiest muscles to develop. They respond quickly to weight work, so you'll see and feel the difference quickly. Besides improving your appearance, strong muscles make your neck less susceptible to injury. This is im-

portant because many weightlifting exercises put stress on the neck. For instance, Bench Press can hurt the neck if you press your head too firmly against the bench as you lift. With any exercise, if you grit your teeth and strain to perform a few more reps, the tension often winds up in your neck. Building a strong neck is a form of injury prevention.

Many shoulder, trap, and chest exercises indirectly work the neck muscles, but they alone aren't enough to build the neck that you need. That's why there are special exercises for the neck. The ones we describe have movements to work the front, back, and sides of your neck.

## NECK EXERCISES

***Wrestler's Bridge*** (illustrated on p. 90)
*Technique:* Use an exercise mat that has about an inch of padding. Lie on your back in the middle of the mat. Bend your knees and pull your feet toward your buttocks until they are flat on the mat; your knees will be bent at about a 90-degree angle. Arch your back and lift your buttocks. Roll most of your body weight onto the top of your head. Slowly roll your head back until your forehead almost touches the mat. Pause, then carefully roll your head forward until your neck touches the mat again. This movement works the muscles at the back of your neck. If you lie face down on the mat instead, you'll target the front and sides of your neck.

NOTE: Be extremely careful when doing this exercise. Keep your legs and feet stable on the mat so that your body weight doesn't stress—and possibly injure—your neck. As you roll your head on the mat to work your neck muscles, do so slowly and cautiously, with no quick, jerky movements. If Wrestler's Bridge feels uncomfortable,

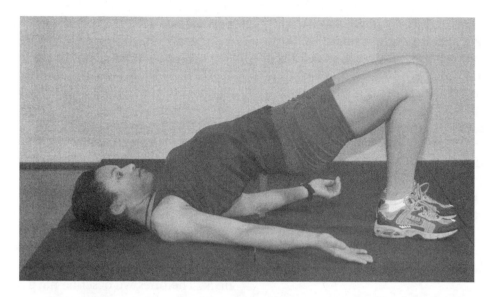

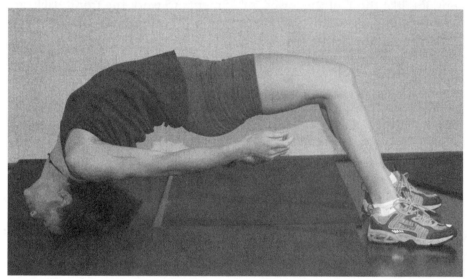

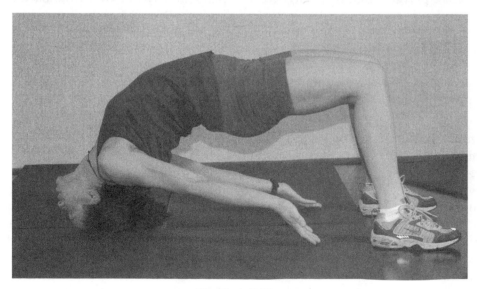

**Wrestler's Bridge**

don't do it. There are other exercises that can work your neck. If you want to do Wrestler's Bridge but don't have an exercise mat, you can place a folded-up towel under your head.

### Hand Pressure with Partner

*Technique:* Lie on your back on a flat bench, with your head hanging off one end. Have a partner stand beside you and place his or her palms on your forehead, perhaps placing a towel between the palms and your forehead. Keeping your body stationary, raise your head forward until your chin touches your chest. As you are raising your head, your partner places gentle pressure on your forehead. This resistance works the neck muscles. After your chin touches your chest, lower your head to the starting position (slightly below the bench) without pressure from your partner. Raise your head again with the person pressing down on your forehead. This resistance works the muscles at the front of your neck. You can also lie face down on the bench. Your partner then presses against the back of your head as you raise your head toward your back. This movement targets the muscles at the back of your neck.

NOTE: For variety, you can lie on your side and have the partner press against the side of your head as you raise it toward your shoulder. With each different movement, you'll feel different parts of your neck at work. As with Wrestler's Bridge, do this exercise cautiously and slowly. Never jerk your head up or down—that places too much stress on your neck. Communicate with your partner so that he or she is not placing too much pressure on your head. You want gentle pressure only.

### Neck Raise Using Weights

*Technique:* This exercise is identical to Hand Pressure with Partner, except that you don't have a partner. Instead, you use weight plates for resistance. Lie on your back on a flat bench, with your head extending off one end. Place a small towel on your forehead, then put a weight plate (no more than 5 or 10 pounds at the beginning) on top of the towel. Grab either side of the weight to keep it in place. Then gradually raise your head until your chin almost touches your chest. Pause, then lower your head until it's below the top of the bench again. You can also lie face down on the bench, or on your side, to work other neck muscles.

NOTE: To avoid injury, *never* use heavy weight for the Neck Raise. The muscles of the neck are fairly easy to develop and don't require heavy weight. Proper form is more important than the amount of weight. You want just enough weight to provide gentle resistance. On all neck exercises, be sure not to strain as much as you do when working other parts of your body.

### Neck Strap

*Technique:* This is one of the oldest neck exercises and one of the best. It requires the use of a neck strap, available at most stores that sell weight-lifting equipment. The strap is made of crisscrossed leather pieces and fits over the top of your head and down the sides. Weights are attached to a chain that dangles from the front of the apparatus. Lie on your chest or back on a flat bench and raise and lower your head. Alternatively, you can lie on your side and lift up the side of your head.

NOTE: Use light weight and perform the movements slowly and carefully.

# 7

## Intermediate Arm Exercises

"The more my biceps stood out, the bigger I wanted them to be. The bigger they became, the more I worked them. Big arms, after all, are the most famous symbol of bodybuilding, more so than any other body part."

—Ronnie Coleman, six-time Mr. Olympia

If you survey top bodybuilders, you will find many reasons why they took up the sport. Obviously, they all wanted to improve their physiques and build bigger muscles overall.

Most people who take up bodybuilding first become infatuated with big arms—specifically biceps. A big pair of biceps—or "guns," as they're sometimes called—stand out like no other muscle group. Big biceps convey power, strength, *authority*.

The muscles of the chest, shoulders, abs, and legs can remain somewhat hidden beneath a bodybuilder's clothes, but massive biceps stand out like two mountain peaks, especially with a short-sleeved shirt. Some beginning weight lifters care only about biceps development. They do curl after curl until their biceps look like cantaloupes. That's okay—if they later apply the same dedication to developing other muscles. Let's face it, a pair of 20-inch biceps looks strange alongside a scrawny chest and skinny legs.

One of the goals of this book is to encourage you to develop your muscles equally—from head to toe.

If you ever hope to compete in bodybuilding contests, you must be well-proportioned, with no glaring weaknesses.

In this chapter, we'll tell you how to develop biceps that will be the envy of others. We'll also cover the other arm muscles—the triceps and the muscles of the forearms—that sometimes get little attention. If you build these muscles as well, your biceps will appear bigger.

We hope you haven't skipped the chapters on other muscle groups to get to this chapter. Arm development is essential—and fun—but it should occur at the same pace that you develop the rest of your body. With that caveat, let's talk about arms.

### BICEPS

"When I began training, I would study photographs of bodybuilders, and what drew my attention most was huge biceps," Arnold Schwarzenegger says. "I would go through the magazines, page by page, looking for examples of outstanding biceps and vow that someday my arms would look like that too."

As Arnold and others learned, building championship biceps is more difficult—and requires more sophistication—than might seem likely. Even people who know almost nothing about weight lifting are often aware of the basic biceps exercise, Curls—but Curls are only one of many exercises that you must do to fully develop this muscle. Every contour of the biceps must be developed to the max if you want to be a contender in a bodybuilding competition. As a result, you have to attack the biceps from numerous angles in your training. Any weakness in biceps development will become apparent in competition because of the many mandatory poses that feature them.

"Peak" refers to the height of your biceps. The biceps must be tall, not just big around. In addition, a biceps with a high peak must also have sharp definition on all sides: The biceps should rise powerfully and be clearly separate from the triceps beneath it.

Some people naturally have big upper arms, even without doing serious weight training. There's a huge difference, however, between having arms that are large and shapeless and having arms that meet the requirements for a bodybuilder—cut and defined, as if sculpted out of marble.

As discussed previously, genetics plays a key role in bodybuilding success. Some people will train much harder than others but still won't have a top-notch physique. Differences in genetics often become apparent in biceps training.

Some bodybuilders have biceps that are naturally tall, but not particularly thick and full. Others have plenty of fullness, but their biceps aren't very tall. These differences are largely the result of genetics and are hard to change.

At the highest levels of bodybuilding, there are few training secrets. If a top competitor realizes he needs taller biceps, he knows the exercises he must do. Still, he may not be able to achieve the height he wants. Should he become discouraged and give up? No.

The biceps is one of many muscles that judges evaluate. Someone with shorter biceps may have an outstanding chest, shoulders, and legs. A bodybuilding title goes to the person with the best overall size and proportion. If you have short biceps, work hard to make them as thick and full as possible. The other dimensions can help make up for biceps that aren't tall.

If you look at photographs of bodybuilding champions over the years, you'll find that not all of them had "perfect" biceps—just as they didn't all have a perfect chest, shoulders, or legs. A bodybuilding champion is the sum of the parts.

Your height plays a key role in how big your biceps appear. People who are short normally have short arms, and it's easier to build biceps that *look* huge if your arms are short. For instance, a pair of 20-inch biceps on someone who is 5'8" looks much bigger than 20-inch biceps on someone who is 6'4". If you're tall, you'll have to develop even bigger biceps to compete against a shorter contender.

Bodybuilders of all heights should do exercises that work the biceps through a full range of motion. It's important not to "cheat" on biceps exercises. If you allow your elbows and shoulders to help you do Curls, for example, your biceps won't get a full workout—especially at the lowest and highest points of each rep. As a result, your biceps won't develop as much as they should.

In the exercises that follow, you'll notice a wide variety of lifting motions. Some of the exercises use a barbell, some use a dumbbell, and some use machines. They are performed standing or sitting, on flat benches or incline benches. Taken together, this array of exercises will help you build biceps that are impressive from any angle, flexed or relaxed.

## TRICEPS

Triceps, the muscles on the back of the upper arms, don't get enough respect. Beginning bodybuilders love to focus on biceps, and some don't even think about working on their triceps. That's a shame. The triceps is actually a larger muscle than the biceps. It isn't as dramatic, but it makes up about two-thirds of the size of the upper arm. As you can see, the best way to increase the circumference of your upper arms is to develop your triceps.

The triceps should have the same degree of definition as the biceps, although that can be difficult to achieve. A fully developed triceps looks somewhat like an upside-down horseshoe. It has two distinct vertical sides and a thicker horizontal slab at the top. It should be distinct from the deltoid muscle above it as well as from the biceps on the front of the arm.

Triceps development requires dedication and commitment. Since it is a more complex muscle than the biceps, you may have to do even more exercises and sets for your triceps than for your biceps. In the upper levels of bodybuilding, it's impossible to hide weak triceps development.

Biceps exercises generally involve bending your upper arm toward your body. Triceps exercises, by contrast, normally require you to straighten your upper arm against resistance. That's how these muscles on the back of your arms get work. You need to pick exercises that target the top, middle, and lower parts of the triceps.

Here again, genetics plays an important role in developing this muscle. Some bodybuilders can build massive triceps fairly easily, while others have to repeatedly "bomb" them to achieve similar results.

Hand position is critical in triceps exercises. A narrow grip on a barbell produces a different effect than a wide grip. With dumbbells, you get different results based on the orientation of your palms. In bodybuilding, little details can make a big difference.

Be aware that some triceps exercises can cause elbow pain. Exercises that bother one person won't necessarily bother another, however, so pay attention to your elbows during and after triceps work. Don't do an exercise that is clearly painful, or you may develop a chronic problem. There are plenty of triceps exercises to choose from that likely won't cause you elbow pain.

## FOREARMS

As a kid, you may have watched the TV cartoon *Popeye*. Remember his forearms? They were massive—ridiculous looking, in fact, and entirely out of proportion to his biceps, which hardly seemed to exist.

Big forearms draw attention—just like big biceps. Visually, they ensure that your lower arm is in proportion to your upper arm. Forearm work can be rewarding, because these muscles often respond quickly to weight training. With the right exercises, you can really pump up your forearms. You'll also be able to create impressive definition.

Forearm strength is also important. Most upper body exercises involve lifting with your forearms. If you don't have the strength to lift heavy weight, other muscle groups can't benefit from the exercise.

Some people incorrectly assume that they don't need to specifically train their forearms. The truth is, even though forearms are involved in most upper body exercises, these exercises don't specifically target the forearms. To achieve a well-developed physique, you must focus on each and every muscle during your training regimen. Forearms are no exception. Make them a priority right from the start.

## EXERCISES

### Biceps

#### *Standing Barbell Curl*

*Technique:* This is the most basic biceps exercise, having been performed by bodybuilders since the sport began. Kneel and grab a barbell with an under-hand grip (palms up, thumbs out) and your hands at shoulder width. Stand up and straighten your arms so that

*Note:* The models are not wearing belts in the photographs in this chapter because they are lifting light weight for demonstration purposes.

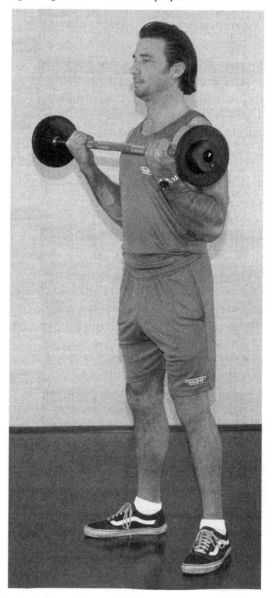

**Standing Barbell Curl**

the barbell rests against your thighs. Your feet should be slightly more than shoulder-width apart. Keep your body stationary and your elbows at your sides, then lift your forearms (and the bar) out, up, and in toward your chest in a wide semicircle. Keep your wrists firm (don't bend them toward your torso) until the very end of the movement. Stop lifting when the bar is at the top of your chest and can't go any higher. Pause, then lower the barbell to the starting position, elbows at your sides.

NOTE: To get maximum benefit from this exercise, it's critical to keep your upper and lower body stationary as you lift. Wear a belt to help stabilize your lower back. Don't let your elbows move in front of your body as you lift, because that shifts some of the work from your biceps to your shoulders. If you can't keep your upper and lower body stationary while performing Curls, you're using too much weight. Proper form is more important than heavy weight. You could even injure your back if you use too much weight and sway back and forth. Advanced bodybuilders sometimes "cheat" (use their backs a little) when lifting very heavy weights. That's okay because they have years of experience and only cheat with a specific goal in mind. As a beginner, stick with strict form. For variety, you can change your grip on the bar. With a grip that's narrower than shoulder width, you'll work your inner biceps more. With a wider grip, you'll place more stress on the outer biceps.

### Arm Blaster

*Technique:* This exercise is identical to the Standing Barbell Curl, except that you use a piece of equipment called an Arm Blaster. It's a metal band, about as wide as a weightlifter's belt, that has a slight S curve at both ends. It rests against your abs, and a strap wraps around your neck to keep it in place. The Arm Blaster has a single purpose: to keep your elbows steady and isolate all the effort on your biceps. It doesn't allow you to cheat nearly as much.

When you use the Arm Blaster for the first time, it may feel odd. You'll probably be surprised at how much more difficult it makes Standing Barbell Curls. This tells you that you've been cheating too much before. When you're using the Arm Blaster, don't cheat with your back and lower body to compensate. At least at first, you won't be able to lift as much weight doing the Standing Barbell Curl when you use this piece of equipment.

NOTE: Many people like to use an EZ curl bar, instead of a regular bar, with an Arm Blaster. EZ curl bars, widely found in gyms, are the same length as a regular bar but are wavy instead of straight. This feature allows your hands to turn in slightly, rather than be in line with each other. This is more comfortable for most people and places less strain on the wrists. An EZ curl bar can be used for all varieties of curls.

### Preacher Curl

*Technique:* This exercise uses a preacher bench, which has a small seat (about the height of a regular flat bench) and an armrest platform about chest-high that slopes down and away from the seat at a 45-degree angle. Sit on the seat and place the backs of your upper arms against the platform. At the bottom of the platform, there's a rack that holds a barbell. Straighten your arms and grab the barbell with an underhand grip and your elbows about shoulder-width apart. Press your chest firmly against the platform for support. Lift the bar out and up in a regular curling motion. Stop when the bar is near your chin and you can't lift it any higher. Pause, then gradually lower the weight to the starting position, until your arms are straight. Don't let the barbell bounce at the bottom.

NOTE: The preacher bench serves the same purpose as the Arm Blaster: It keeps your elbows stable and helps prevent you from cheating. The preacher bench is a favorite of many top bodybuilders. In particular, it helps develop the lower biceps near the elbow. Use a light enough weight so that you can keep your arms firmly against the pad without rocking your body. Preacher Curls are normally done with an EZ curl bar.

### Incline Dumbbell Curl

*Technique:* Sit on an incline bench. Grab a dumbbell in each hand. Let your arms hang loosely down. Keep your elbows close to your sides and slightly in front of your torso. Slowly lift both dumbbells at the same time in the regular curling motion, stopping when your arms can't go any higher. Keep your upper arms steady as you lift. At the top, pause, then lower the dumbbells to the starting position. At the bottom, stop for an extra count before lifting the dumbbells again. This will keep you from relying on momentum to swing the dumbbells up, thereby making the exercise too easy. The Incline Dumbbell Curl is also designed to minimize cheating.

NOTE: Try rotating your wrists slightly outward as you lift. Start with your palms up, then gradually rotate

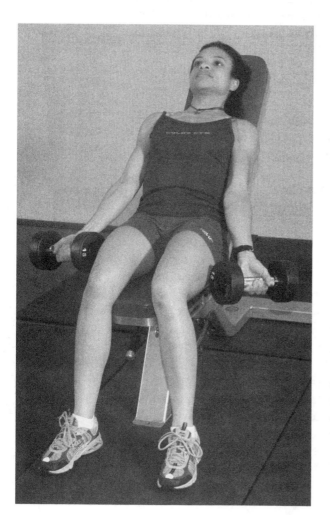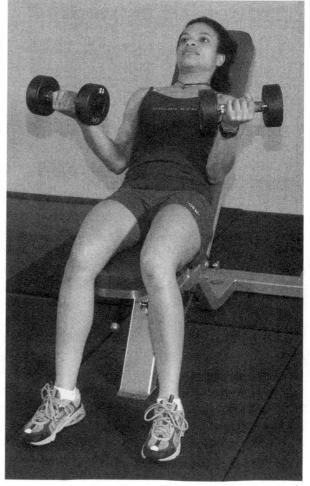

**Incline Dumbbell Curl**

your wrists so that your palms are turned out at the top. As you lower the dumbbells, rotate your wrists back so that your palms are oriented up again at the bottom. Many bodybuilders find that this wrist rotation produces a higher "peak" to the biceps, as well as creating better overall size and definition.

### Seated Dumbbell Curl

*Technique:* This exercise is identical to the Incline Dumbbell Curl, except that you sit on a flat bench. As a result, your back won't be as stable and you may have to fight a tendency to cheat. However, by sitting erect, instead of leaning against an incline bench, you work your biceps at a slightly different angle. Variety is always good in arm workouts.

NOTE: You'll get more benefit if you rotate your wrists during the movement, as described above for the Incline Dumbbell Curl. Start with your palms up, then rotate your wrists so your palms are turned out at the top. You can raise the dumbbells either one at a time or simultaneously. If you lift them one at a time, raise one arm just as the other arm reaches the lowest position; this helps create a smooth rhythm as you lift.

### Hammer Curl (illustrated on p. 100)

*Technique:* This exercise is identical to the Seated Dumbbell Curl, except that you start with your palms turned

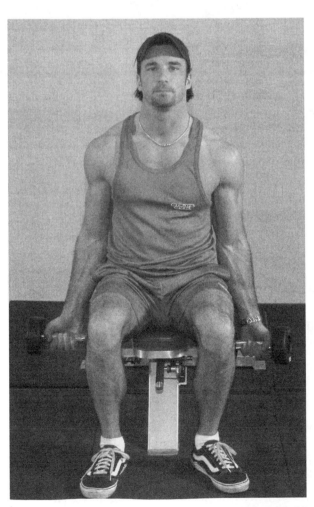
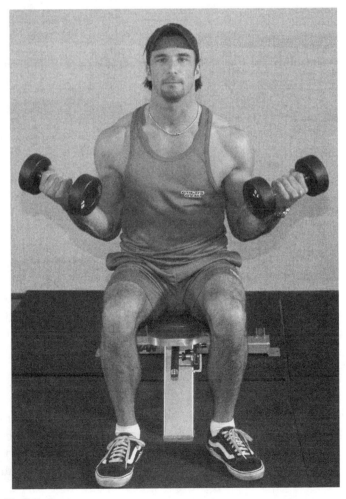

**Seated Dumbbell Curl**

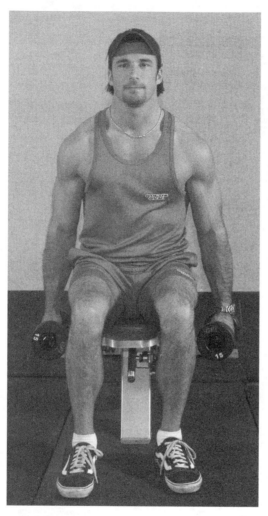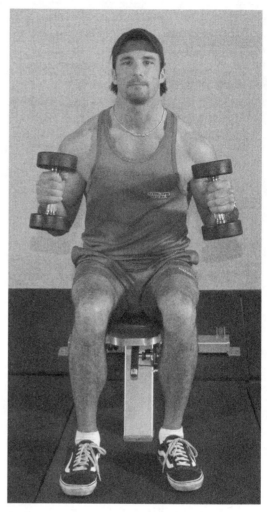

**Hammer Curl**

inward and keep them in that position throughout the movement. You don't rotate your wrists.

NOTE: By keeping your palms facing inward throughout, you work your forearm muscles as well as the biceps. You can do the Hammer Curl seated or standing. Either way, keep your elbows close to your sides and your upper arms stable. You may lift your arms either one at a time or simultaneously.

### Concentration Curl

*Technique:* This is an excellent exercise for adding height to your biceps. Sit on the end of a flat bench with your legs apart. Grab a dumbbell in your right hand. Lean your torso forward until your back is at a 45-degree angle.

Place your right elbow against the inside of your right thigh. Straighten your arm with the dumbbell near the floor. Gradually raise the weight toward your shoulder, keeping your elbow pressed against the inside of your thigh for support. At the top, pause, then lower the dumbbell to the starting position. After you finish the reps, lift with your left arm.

NOTE: When you're lifting with your right arm, place your left hand on the side of your left thigh or your forearm on top of the thigh (and vice versa). This will help keep your upper body stationary and the effort focused on your biceps. The key to this exercise is concentrating all the work on your biceps.

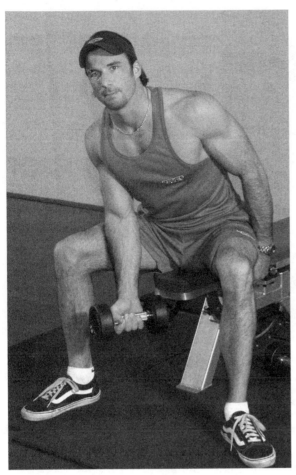
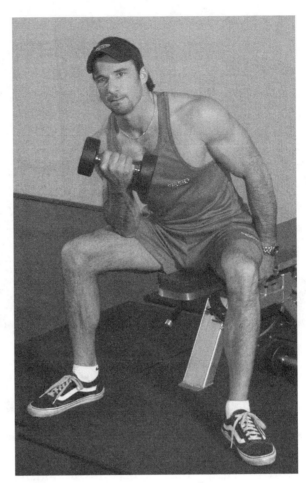

**Concentration Curl**

***Lying Dumbbell Curl*** (illustrated on p. 102)

*Technique:* The Lying Dumbbell Curl is a variation of the Seated Dumbbell Curl, described above. It allows you to more fully stretch your biceps, lengthening the muscle and improving its appearance. Lie on your back on a flat bench, with your knees off the end of the bench and your feet on the floor for stability. Grab a dumbbell in each hand. Let your arms hang loosely down. Hold the dumbbells about an inch off the floor, with your elbows slightly bent. Slowly lift both dumbbells toward your shoulders at the same time, using a regular curling motion. Keep your elbows close to your sides and your upper arms stationary. Raise the dumbbells as high as possible, then pause and lower them until your arms are almost straight.

NOTE: Don't lock your elbows at the bottom. That removes some of the tension from the biceps, and it lets them rest momentarily. You may not be able to use as much weight on this exercise as you can with the Seated Dumbbell Curl. That's because you're lying on your back, and your biceps are working against gravity more as they lift the weight. You can raise your head and shoulders a few inches off the bench if it makes the movement more comfortable. Just don't let your head and shoulders sway to help you lift the weight.

**Cable Curl**

*Technique:* For this exercise, you use a machine with a floor-level pulley and cable and with a short horizontal bar (2 to 3 feet long) attached to the

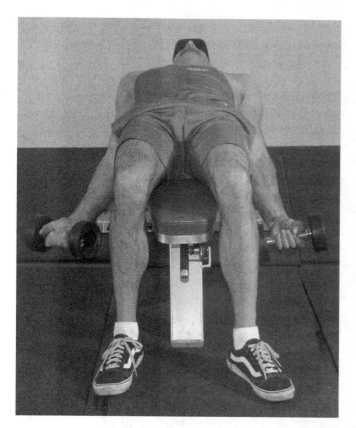 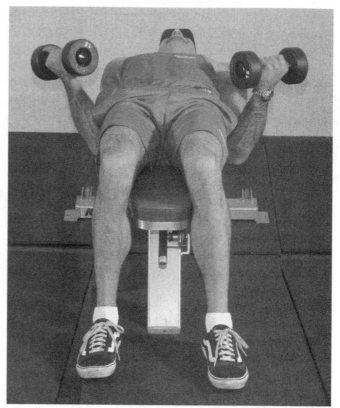

**Lying Dumbbell Curl**

cable. Grab the bar with an underhand grip and with your hands shoulder-width apart. Hold the handle in front of your thighs—just as you would a barbell for the Standing Barbell Curl. The cable should be taut. Lift the handle out and up toward your chest in a wide arc. Keep your elbows close to your side and your upper arms stationary. This is the same lifting motion used for the Standing Barbell Curl.

NOTE: Lean your torso back slightly as you lift to keep the cable taut, but don't let your upper body sway. Because the cable provides continuous tension, there's as much resistance when you lower the weights as when you raise them. This is different from similar exercises with a barbell or dumbbells, where it's easier to lower the weights than to raise them. For variety, you can stand farther away from the weight stack and raise the bar only to your abs instead of to your upper chest.

### Biceps Machine

*Technique:* Most gyms have machines specifically designed to work the biceps. They may vary in appearance, but they provide the same basic lifting motion, using a weight stack for resistance. They have a seat, which is usually adjustable, about the height of a regular flat bench, and some have a back to lean against. Straighten your arms in front of you, parallel to the floor, and place your elbows on the chest-high pad. Grab a handle with each hand (palms up, thumbs out). Lift the handles toward your chest simultaneously, keeping your elbows on the pad. Hold for a moment, then return to the starting position. Repeat.

NOTE: On some biceps machines, you extend your arms straight in front of you, as described above. On others, you extend your arms slightly toward the floor. On the latter machines, the backs of your upper arms rest

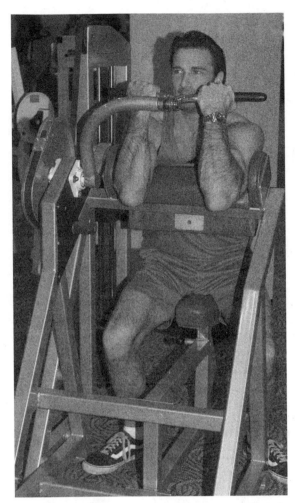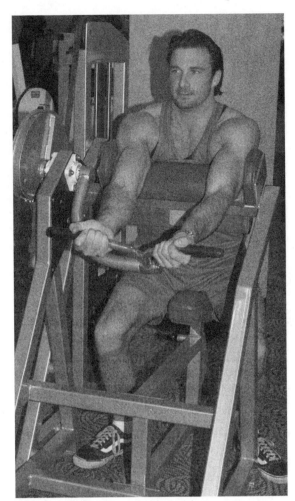

**Biceps Machine**

against a platform that slopes down at about a 45-degree angle. A machine like this simulates the motion of the Preacher Curl.

### Close-Grip Chin-Up (illustrated on pp. 104–105)

*Technique:* Chin-Ups, like Dips, don't use weight. They rely entirely on your body weight for resistance. Stand beneath a horizontal chin-up bar (normally about a foot above your head). Reach up and grab the bar with an underhand grip and with your hands 4 to 6 inches apart. (If the bar is too high, you may have to stand on a stool.) Bend your knees and cross your ankles to keep your lower body stable. Start with your arms almost fully extended and your body hanging under

the bar. Then gradually pull yourself up until your chin is just above the bar. Pause, then carefully lower yourself to the starting position with your arms not quite straight when you reach the lowest point.

NOTE: Don't sway or swing your body up to help you get to the top—this robs the biceps of the full effect. Tilt your torso back slightly as you lift yourself for a smoother movement. You can try placing your hands closer and closer together, even to the point that they touch. A narrow grip works your biceps, whereas a wide grip benefits your lats and other back muscles. Chin-Ups, as you can see, are a very versatile exercise. You can also do this exercise with an overhand grip.

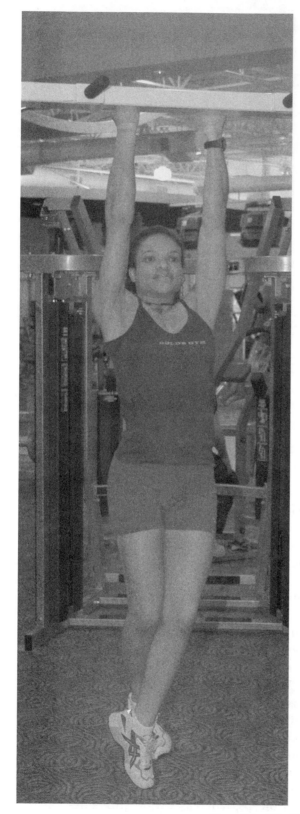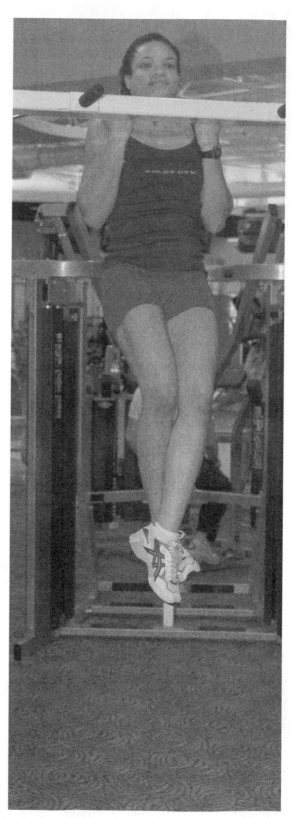

**Close-Grip Chin-Up (underhand grip)**

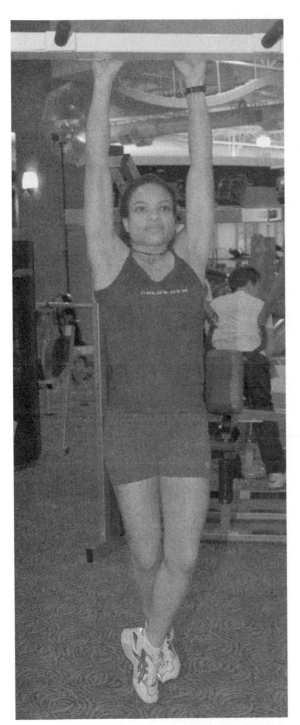
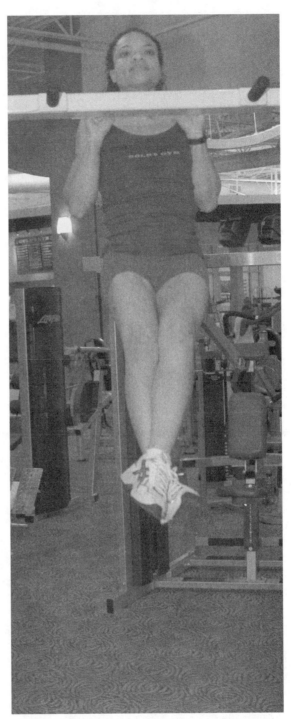

**Close-Grip Chin-Up (overhand grip)**

### Triceps

#### Cable Pressdown

*Technique:* Stand next to a machine with an overhead pulley and cable. Grab the horizontal bar attached to the end of the cable (it may be at eye level or slightly above your head) with an overhand grip. Place your hands 6 to 10 inches apart on the bar and your feet 6 to 10 inches apart. Hold the bar about a foot in front of your torso and even with your chest. With your elbows tucked against your sides, press down on the bar with your lower arms until it touches your thighs and your arms are straight. Keep your upper arms stable. Pause, then let the bar slowly return to a point even with your chest.

NOTE: Keep your torso straight or leaning slightly forward. Don't tilt forward so much that you use your body to press down on the weights. Maintain steady tension on the cable as you raise and lower the weight stack. Keep your elbows even with your torso—don't let them move forward or backward. A variety of bars can be used for the Cable Pressdown; they may be long, short, or in an inverted V shape.

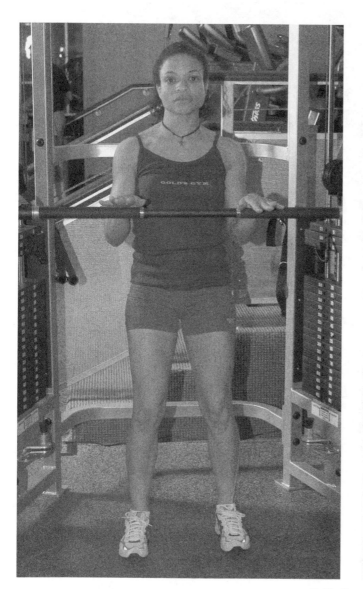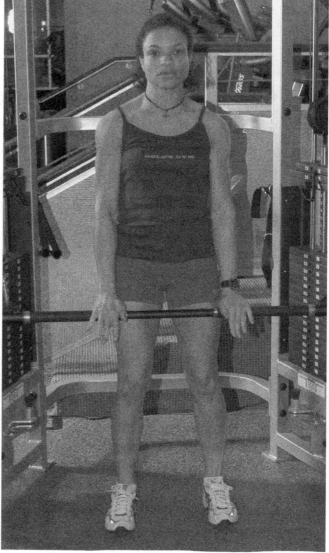

**Cable Pressdown**

*Variations:* There are several variations of the Cable Pressdown:

- You can use an Arm Blaster, described in the Biceps section above. This metal band rests in front of your abs and keeps your elbows in place, forcing you to do the Cable Pressdown with very strict form.
- You can lie on an incline bench, with your back to the weight stack. Grab the bar over your head and lower it into position in front of your collarbone. With this as the starting point, press down on the bar until it touches the tops of your thighs.
- You can do the Cable Pressdown with an underhand grip (palms up, thumbs out) to work the triceps from a different angle. This can be done standing or seated.
- You can press down with one arm at a time. To do this, remove the horizontal bar from the cable and replace it with a handle suitable for one hand.

### Seated Triceps Barbell Press

*Technique:* Sit on a flat bench and hold a barbell in front of your chest with an overhand grip—as if you're preparing to press the bar overhead. Carefully lift the barbell over your head and lower it until it's even with the base of your neck in the back. Bring your hands together on the bar until they are only 3 to 4 inches apart. With your arms bent at a 90-degree angle and your elbows on either side of your head, press the barbell up until your arms straighten overhead. Keep your elbows and upper arms steady. Lower the barbell back to the base of your neck.

NOTE: You can also do this exercise standing, although there's more of a tendency to cheat in that position. For variety or increased comfort, you may do this exercise with an EZ curl bar or on an incline bench.

### Seated Triceps Dumbbell Press

*Technique:* This exercise is identical to the Seated Triceps Barbell Press, except that you use dumbbells. As with all dumbbell exercises, there is a longer range of motion. You can lift either two dumbbells simultaneously or one at a time. Hold the dumbbell(s) behind your head with your palm(s) facing up and the bar(s) parallel to the floor. If you are using one dumbbell, you can place both hands on it, holding the bar perpendicular to the floor and with your palms facing inward. Raise the dumbbell(s) straight up, but stop short of locking your elbows. Hold for a moment, then lower the dumbbell(s) to the starting position. Keep your elbows close to your head as you lift.

NOTE: If you lift one dumbbell at a time, place the nonlifting arm across your chest to stabilize your torso. As you lift, keep the dumbbells behind your head—not over your shoulders; this makes your triceps work harder. You may want to do the Seated Triceps Dumbbell Press in front of a mirror in order to check the position of your hands and arms. Don't use too much weight or you could injure your elbow. Perform the motion slowly, without bouncing the weight at the lowest point.

### Lying Barbell Extension (illustrated on p. 108)

*Technique:* Lie on your back on a flat bench, with your head just off one end. Bend your knees so that your feet are on the floor. Hold a barbell behind your head. Bend your arms so that the barbell is near the floor. Keeping your elbows close to your head, lift your forearms (and the bar) straight up. Stop when your hands are above the back of your head (not your forehead). Stop just short of locking your elbows, in order to keep constant tension on your triceps.

NOTE: Lift with a smooth motion,

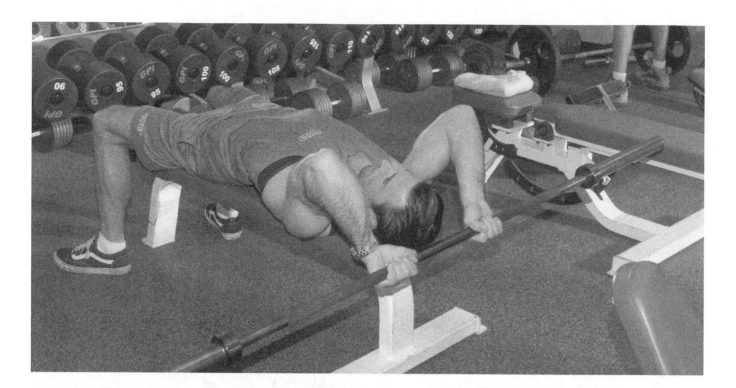

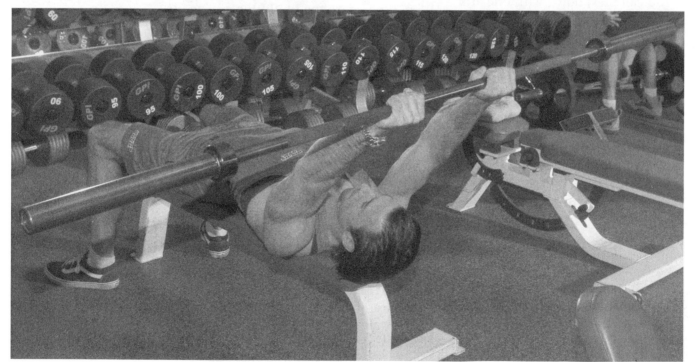

**Lying Barbell Extension**

keeping control of the bar at all times. Don't let it fall quickly as you lower the weight. Start with light weight until you get comfortable with the motion. Be sure to keep your head slightly off one end; this lets you lower the bar farther and get greater extension of your triceps.

*Variations:* There are several variations of the Lying Barbell Extension:

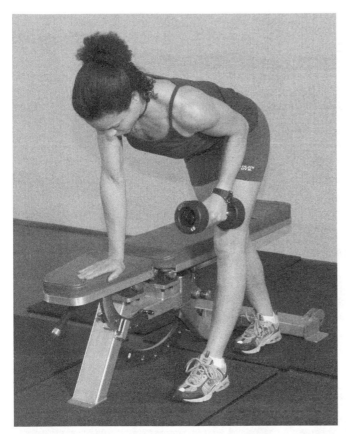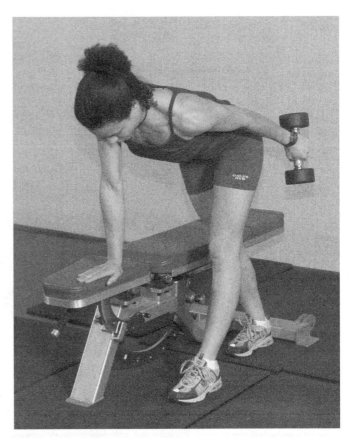

**Dumbbell Kickback**

- Use an EZ curl bar and/or an incline bench.
- Vary the width of your grip on the bar.
- Use dumbbells instead of a barbell. If you do, keep your palms turned inward as you lift.

### Dumbbell Kickback

*Technique:* Stand beside a flat bench. Place your left foot in front of your right. Grab a dumbbell in your left hand and bend your torso so that it's parallel to the floor. Place your right hand on the bench for support. Hold the dumbbell by your left knee, with your elbow bent at a 90-degree angle and your forearm parallel to the floor. Your palm should face inward. Keep your elbow stationary, then press the dumbbell backward until your arm is straight. The dumbbell will be behind your buttocks. Pause, then lower the dumbbell back to the starting position by your knees. When you've finished your reps, repeat the exercise with your right arm, placing your left hand on the bench.

NOTE: Don't swing the weight up. Lift it gradually, feeling your triceps at work. By using a bench for support and positioning one leg in front of the other, you should be able to isolate your triceps.

### Narrow-Grip Bench Press (illustrated on p. 110)

*Technique:* This exercise is identical to the regular Bench Press, except that your hands are much closer together. With Bench Press, your hands are shoulder-width apart in order to benefit your chest and shoulder muscles. To turn Bench Press into a triceps exercise, place your hands only 4 to 6 inches apart on the bar. The lifting and lower-

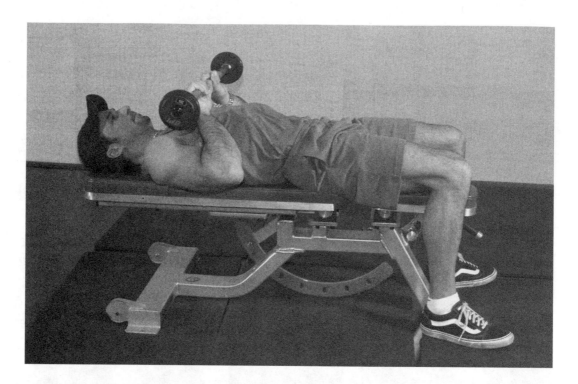

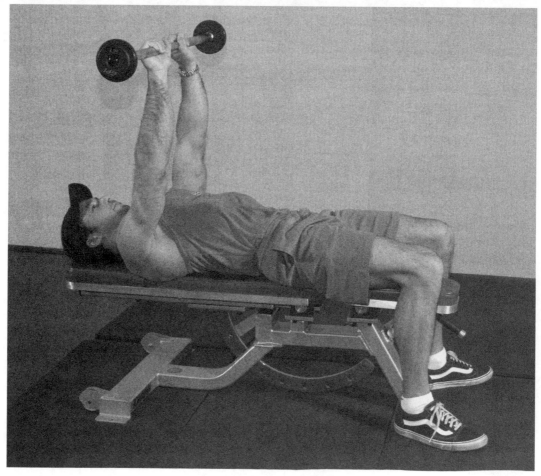

**Narrow-Grip Bench Press**

ing motion is the same as with Bench Press.

**NOTE:** When you lift the barbell off the supports to begin the exercise, use a normal overhand grip, with your hands shoulder-width apart. This will help you more easily control and balance the bar. Once it's comfortably overhead, you can move your hands closer together, then lift and lower the barbell. For variety, you may do this exercise on an incline or decline bench. Regardless of which bench you use, keep your back firmly in place as you lift. Don't arch your back to help you lift the weight. You can also use an EZ curl bar for performing the Narrow-Grip Bench Press; this may reduce the strain on your wrists.

### Triceps Machine

*Technique:* Most gyms have triceps machines, which are very similar to biceps machines. They typically have an adjustable seat about the height of a regular flat bench, and there may be a back to lean against. Rest your elbows on the pad. Bend your arms at the elbow so that your hands are near your face. Grab the two handles with your palms turned inward. Gradually press out and down on the handles until your arms straighten. Pause, then bend your elbows and let the handles slowly return to the starting position near your face. You should feel resistance through the entire movement.

**NOTE:** These machines vary widely in appearance but perform basically

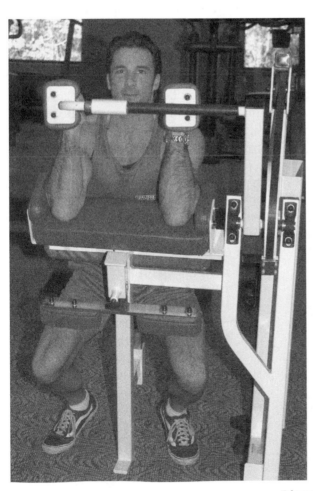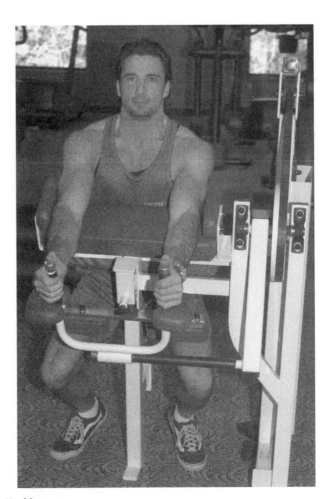

**Triceps Machine**

the same movement. They're effective because they isolate the triceps, making it harder to cheat. They also provide continuous resistance as you raise and lower the weight.

### Long Cable Extension

*Technique:* This exercise uses a cable machine with an overhead pulley. Stand with your back to the weight stack. Reach over your head and grab the horizontal bar with an overhand grip. (Use a short bar if one is available.) Take about three or four steps away from the weight stack, and place one foot in front of the other for stability. Lean forward at the waist at about a 45-degree angle. Make sure the cable is taut. Keep your elbows by your head, your forearms parallel to the floor, and the bar near the back of your neck. Keeping your body stationary, press up and out on the bar until your arms straighten above your head. Look down at the floor and hold, then gradually bend your elbows and let the weight return to the starting position.

NOTE: Use light weight until you get a feel for this exercise and can maintain a comfortable stance and keep your balance. The Long Cable Extension is similar to the Cable Pressdown, described above. The main differences are that, with the Long Cable Extension, you face away from the weight stack and you tilt your torso.

### Dips

*Technique:* Dips were discussed earlier in this book. They are an extremely versatile exercise, but are usually thought to benefit the chest muscles. By changing your body position, however, you can work the triceps very effectively. Normally, you want to lean forward slightly as you lift and lower your body on Dips, but if you keep your torso straight up and down, the stress is shifted to your triceps.

Be sure to bend your knees and cross your ankles in order to keep your legs stable. Lock your elbows at the top and lower yourself until your chest is even with the top of the bars.

NOTE: If you have trouble with Dips, don't lower yourself all the way down at first; otherwise, you'll risk straining your shoulders. Some dip bars have horizontal bars that are parallel, while others taper in at one end. If you use the latter type, try different grip positions on the bars.

*Variation:* Once you become adept at Dips, you can change the position of your hands on the bars to make the exercise much more difficult. Instead of having your palms turned inward, place them so that they are turned outward. This makes your triceps do even more work as you raise and lower your body. In addition, your chest muscles don't come into play nearly as much. However, be very careful with this reverse grip. It should only be used by advanced bodybuilders, because it places much more strain on the wrists and elbows and can therefore lead to injury. If you are uncomfortable or feel unsteady, don't do it. Go back to the normal grip, with your palms turned inward. You can attach weights to your waist for extra resistance.

### Dips Behind Back

*Technique:* In this exercise, you perform a "dipping" motion without using Dip bars. Instead, you use two flat benches, placed parallel to each other and about 4 feet apart. Put your heels on one bench and your palms on the other. Your body will be suspended in the shape of an L—legs parallel to the floor and torso erect. Your buttocks will be just in front of the rear bench and your arms will be straight up and down. From this starting position, gradually bend your elbows and lower your buttocks toward the floor. Your heels should remain stationary on the

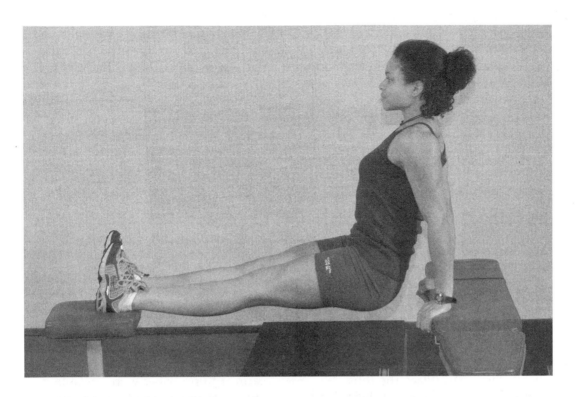

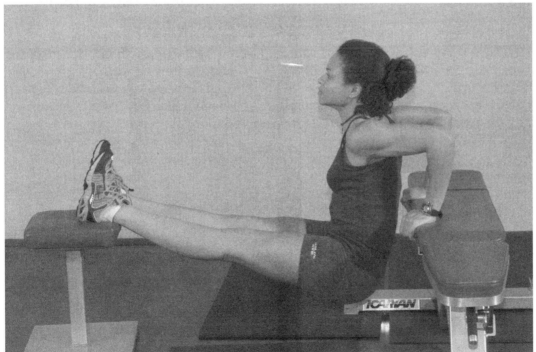

**Dips Behind Back**

front bench as your legs angle down. Stop when your buttocks are a few inches off the floor. Don't lower yourself farther than feels comfortable. Pause, then gradually straighten your arms and raise your torso until your legs are parallel to the floor again.

NOTE: Keep your feet stable on the front bench throughout the motion. Make sure you maintain control of your body so that you don't suddenly fall to the floor. Dips Behind Back places considerable strain on your elbows, so do it carefully. Done properly, it's one of the best triceps exercises. For variety, you can change the placement of your hands on the bench in order to work different parts of the triceps. For extra resistance, you can place a weight on your thighs or have a partner press down gently on your shoulders. At first, however, there's no need for more resistance.

### Forearms

#### Wrist Curl

*Technique:* Sit on the end of a flat bench with your feet shoulder-width apart. Grab a barbell with an underhand grip and your hands only 2 to 3 inches apart. Place the tops of your forearms on your thighs, with your forearms angling in slightly. Your wrists and the barbell should hang slightly beyond your knees. Bend your wrists down so that the tops of your hands touch your kneecaps. Let the barbell roll from your palms onto your fingers—this is the starting point. Now lift your wrists up toward your body, keeping your forearms against your thighs. As you bend your wrists, let the barbell roll back onto your palms. Stop when your wrists won't go any higher. Your knuckles will be turned upward. Pause, then gradually bend your wrists down and lower the barbell again.

NOTE: Start with light weight until you get the feel for this exercise. With such a narrow grip, it takes practice to keep the bar in balance as you raise and lower it. Be sure to keep your wrists beyond your knees and your forearms steady throughout. By moving only your wrists, you isolate your forearm muscles. If you move your entire arm, you get help from other muscles. For variety, you can try a wider grip on the bar. Expect your forearm muscles to

burn as you perform the barbell Wrist Curl, especially at first. That's a sign that you're doing it correctly and making progress. Add weight gradually so that you don't strain your wrists. Wrists are vital for almost all weightlifting exercises—don't risk injuring them.

*Variations:* These modifications will work the forearm muscles in slightly different ways, improving their development.

- Reverse your grip. Grab the barbell with an overhand grip (palms down, thumbs in) instead of an underhand grip. Widen your grip so that your hands are 6 to 8 inches apart. Otherwise, perform Wrist Curls as described above. This grip focuses more effort on the muscles on top of your forearm. You probably won't be able to use as much weight as you can with an underhand grip.
- Stand and hold the barbell behind you, against your buttocks, with your hands shoulder-width apart and your palms turned away from your body. Your thumbs should rest against the sides of your thighs. Let the barbell roll from your palms onto your fingers as described above. At the lowest point, your wrists will be in a straight line with your forearms. Then bend your wrists up, keeping your forearms stationary, to raise the weight. The barbell will roll back onto your palms.
- Sit on a preacher bench and place your forearms on the angled armrest platform. Grip a barbell with an overhand grip and your hands about 8 inches apart. Start with your palms turned toward the floor and your wrists in a straight line with your forearms. Bend your wrists up and toward your body so that your palms turn outward.
- Use dumbbells instead of a barbell. Many people prefer dumbbells

for Wrist Curls because they place less strain on the wrists and they allow a longer range of motion. Sit on the end of a flat bench with your forearms on your thighs and your hands extending beyond your knees. Curl the dumbbells toward you as you would with a barbell. Start with an underhand grip, but you can also try an overhand grip. You can lift with both arms simultaneously or with one at a time.

### Reverse Barbell Curl

*Technique:* This exercise involves your arms, not just your wrists. It is identical to the Standing Barbell Curl for biceps, except that you use an overhand grip instead of an underhand grip. That slight difference transforms it into a forearm exercise. Stand with your feet slightly more than shoulder-width apart. Grab a barbell with an overhand grip and with your hands shoulder-width apart. Straighten your

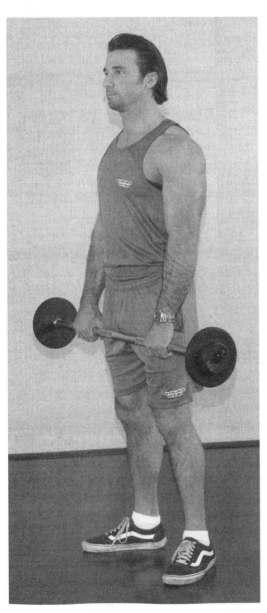
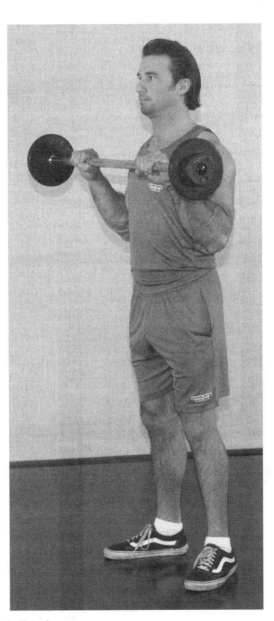

**Reverse Barbell Curl**

arms, holding the barbell against your thighs. Lift your forearms out, up, and in toward your body in a wide arc. Keep your wrists firm and your elbows at your sides. Stop when the bar almost touches your chest. Pause, then lower the weight along the same path to the starting position.

NOTE: Don't use as much weight for the Reverse Barbell Curl as you do for the Standing Barbell Curl. (Your forearm muscles are not as strong as your biceps.) Keep your upper and lower body stationary as you lift and lower the bar. Wear a belt to stabilize your lower back. Don't let your elbows move in front of or behind your torso. For variety, you can do the Reverse Barbell Curl on a preacher bench or you can use an EZ curl bar.

### Reverse Cable Curl

*Technique:* This exercise is identical to the Reverse Barbell Curl, except that you use a machine with a floor-level pulley. With an overhand grip, hold the handle against your thighs. Lean back slightly to keep the cable taut. Then raise and lower your forearms in the same manner as described above.

### Hammer Curl (illustrated on p. 100)

*Technique:* We included the Hammer Curl in the biceps section, but it's equally good for forearm development. It works the upper forearm muscles where they join the biceps. Either standing or seated, hold a dumbbell at your side, with your palm turned inward and your thumb on top, and

your arm hanging straight down— this is the starting position. Raise your forearm out, up, and in toward your body, stopping when you can't raise it any higher. Keep your wrist firm throughout.

NOTE: Keep your elbows at your sides and your upper arms stable. You can also use a dumbbell in each hand, lifting your arms one at a time or simultaneously. If you sit, you can use a flat bench or an incline bench.

### Zottman Curl

*Technique:* The Zottman Curl is similar to the Hammer Curl. Hold a dumbbell in your right hand with your palm turned up and your arm hanging straight down. Lift the dumbbell straight up toward your right shoulder. About halfway up, rotate your wrist 180 degrees so that your palm turns downward. Stop when your right hand reaches your shoulder. Keep your elbow at your right side. Hold, then lower the weight, rotating your wrist 180 degrees back so that your palm turns up again as your arm returns to your right side.

NOTE: Zottman Curls aren't commonly done today, but they're very effective for forearm development. At the beginning of the exercise, you work the muscles on the bottom of your forearm. After you rotate your wrist, your upper forearm muscles come into play. You can lift one arm at a time for several reps or you can alternate arms as you do each rep.

# 8

# Intermediate Leg Exercises

"My leg workout is the most intense of any body part. It takes a lot of hard work and totally drains me. On the morning of my workout, I am totally preoccupied with it. I can't think of anything else."

—Nimrod King, former top bodybuilder

Beginning bodybuilders want big arms. They wouldn't mind broad shoulders and a thick chest too. And "six-pack" abs would be swell too.

Unfortunately, many aspiring bodybuilders don't give any thought to their legs. Maybe they figure their legs don't show under their clothing, so why bother to develop them? Maybe they think that their thighs and calves get enough work during everyday activity and on the treadmill. Maybe they tried weight training for their legs once and thought it was too hard.

Whatever the reason, avoiding leg work is a bad idea. Too often, you see people who have huge arms, massive upper bodies—and tiny legs. It looks like they've never done a leg exercise in their lives. And that may be the case.

Even some bodybuilding stars admit that they didn't focus on their legs as beginners. "I made the classic mistake of training to build a showy upper body while neglecting my leg development," says Lou Ferrigno, a bodybuilding champ of the 1970s who starred in the TV series *The Incredible Hulk.* "Later,

I realized that if I was to succeed as a bodybuilder, I'd need to bring my legs into balance with my upper body. I also knew that it would be tough sledding to accomplish this transformation because my upper body had exploded in growth."

Some people simply dislike doing leg exercises—Squats, Leg Extensions, and Leg Presses are strenuous, and even painful. It takes mental, as well as physical, strength to stick with them. Yet serious bodybuilders don't avoid leg work, because they know they can't afford to. Today's events are so competitive that well-developed legs can provide the winning margin. Contestants realize that they must spend hours and hours training their thighs and calves.

It can be frustrating to train your legs. Some people, because of their genetic makeup, struggle to make significant gains, particularly in their calves. Even Arnold Schwarzenegger fell into that category. He says that in his early years, he never allowed his calves to be photographed. They were so underdeveloped that he thought they would detract from the well-developed arms, shoulders, and chest that he loved to show off. In his book *The New Encyclopedia of Modern Bodybuilding,* Arnold has a photo that shows him posing in knee-deep water. His calves aren't even visible!

Today, he can laugh about such self-consciousness. After years of determined training, he finally developed his calves to the extraordinary level of the rest of his physique—but it wasn't easy, and it may not be easy for you. That's no excuse for avoiding leg training. Your thigh muscles are the largest of your entire body. You can't simply "write off" such a significant muscle group.

Think of your legs as pillars. You don't want skinny, weak pillars trying to support an otherwise impressive physique.

You may be surprised to find that your legs respond well to weight training. Tom Platz, a top bodybuilder of the 1960s and '70s, developed enormous thighs, measuring 28 inches in circumference. He loved leg work and trained harder than most, but he also had the benefit of good genes. His thighs developed faster and became much bigger than those of other bodybuilders who trained in much the same manner.

You may have similar potential. You'll never know until you seriously train your legs. Bodybuilding champs normally have one muscle group that stands out above the rest—whether it's arms, chest, back, abs, or legs. Your legs may turn out to be your best attribute.

To get maximum results with leg exercises, you have to work up to using heavy weight and doing many, many sets. You need the intensity to do a few more reps when you feel like your legs are about to give out.

"I accepted the fact that leg workouts simply have to be brutal to be effective," Schwarzenegger says.

"Normal workouts are hard enough, but if thighs happen to be a weak point in your physique, you have to be prepared to push yourself even more. That means forcing yourself to break down any inhibition or barrier, blasting your thighs to create total development."

Paul DeMayo, a modern-day champion, agrees. "If you want to make progress in your leg training . . . your mind has to be into it," he says. "Most people with underdeveloped legs dread leg training because they know if it's done right, it'll take the life out of you. So a lot of people avoid the hard work. You have to be willing to put forth the maximum effort.

"Legs are the basis of your upper body strength. They have to support you during all standing exercises. They are the source of your drive and speed in all sports."

Because leg exercises can be so strenuous and often involve heavy weight, you should have a spotter or a training partner nearby. You never want to run the risk of taking too much weight and being unable to handle it. This is especially true when doing Squats with a barbell. Bodybuilders have been known to seriously injure their backs or knees by trying to squat with too much weight.

## EXERCISES

### Thighs

*Squats* (illustrated on p. 31)

*Technique:* Squats are the tried-and-true exercise for thigh development. They are like Bench Press for the chest and the Standing Barbell Curl for the biceps. No bodybuilding champ has ever developed his thighs without doing hours and hours of Squats. They can, however, be dangerous if done improperly. You *must* learn proper form before tackling even moderate weight.

To start the exercise, turn your back toward a barbell on a shoulder-height rack. (This is far safer than lifting a heavy barbell off the floor and putting it on your shoulders.) Bend your knees and get under the bar so that it lies across the back of your shoulders. Grab it with an overhand grip and with your hands slightly more than shoulder-width apart. Make sure you have a firm grip, then straighten your legs to lift the bar off the rack. Take a few steps forward. Be sure the bar is balanced properly before proceeding. Place your feet slightly more than shoulder-width apart and bend your knees a little. While keeping your back straight, bend your knees fully and lower yourself until your thighs are just lower than parallel to the floor. At the bottom, pause and be sure you have a firm grip on the bar and a stable stance. Then gradually stand up, keeping the barbell steady on your shoulders. Don't bounce at the bottom to make standing easier. Let your thigh muscles do all the work.

NOTE: Wear a belt to support your lower back and have a spotter nearby for safety. It should go without saying, but make sure the collars are secured on the bar before beginning. You don't want weights to fall off, injuring you or someone else. As you lower yourself and stand up again, always keep your head up and your eyes looking forward. This helps stabilize your lower back and avoid injury. Make sure the bar stays directly in line with your feet throughout the movement. In the beginning, use light weight. As you gain experience, you can add weight and try to lower yourself farther—past the point where your thighs are parallel to the floor. However, do so cautiously. Some advanced bodybuilders go down so far that their buttocks touch their ankles, but this can place enormous strain on your knees and back if you're not prepared.

*Variations:* Squats are normally done with your feet shoulder-width apart and your toes pointing out slightly. If you widen the stance, you work your inner thighs more. If you turn your toes in, your inner thighs get even more work. A narrower stance focuses effort on the outer thighs.

### Smith Machine Squat

*Technique:* A Smith Machine has a large rack that supports a barbell and vertical rails that let it slide up and down along a fixed path as you perform Squats. The benefits of using a Smith Machine are that you don't have to balance the barbell on your shoulders, and you don't have to fear taking too much weight and not being able stand up with it. A Smith Machine holds the barbell in place and allows you to get out from under it. For beginners, particularly, this machine is good because it gives a feel for the squatting motion while relieving fears of being injured.

NOTE: Even some advanced bodybuilders do Squats on a Smith Machine. That's fine, particularly if a person has knee or back problems. However, your thighs will get more benefit if you can handle using a regular barbell instead, because balancing full weight on your shoulders forces your thighs to work harder.

### Dumbbell Squat (illustrated on p. 120)

*Technique:* The Dumbbell Squat is a good exercise for beginners. It involves the standard squatting motion, but you hold a dumbbell in each hand at your sides instead of having a barbell on your shoulders. With dumbbells, you don't have to worry about taking too much weight. If you do, you can simply set the dumbbells on the floor. Hold the dumbbells with your palms turned inward.

NOTE: Dumbbell Squats allow you to get used to the squatting motion.

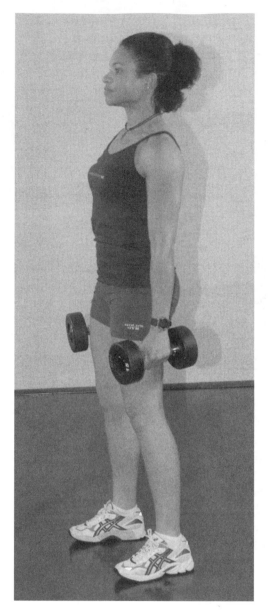

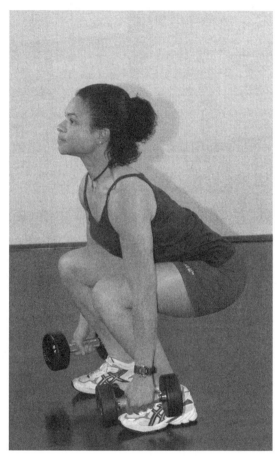

**Dumbbell Squat**

Once you gain confidence, you can move up to using a barbell or a Smith Machine. The drawback to doing this exercise with dumbbells is that you can't hold enough weight to build massive thighs.

### Front Squat

*Technique:* This exercise is identical to regular Squats, except that you hold the barbell *in front of* your neck instead of behind it. Face a barbell on a shoulder-height rack. Bend your knees

slightly so that you can lower your chest under the bar. Grab the bar with a wide overhand grip. Carefully straighten your legs to lift the barbell off the rack. It should lie at the base of your neck and rest across your deltoids. Take a few steps away from the rack. Make sure you have a firm grasp and a steady stance, then perform the normal squatting motion.

NOTE: You may want to place a towel underneath the bar to make it more comfortable and secure against your neck and delts. With Front Squats, you won't be able to use as much weight, because your buttocks don't assist, as they do when the bar is behind your neck. Some people prefer to do this exercise with a different grip altogether, as shown in the accompanying photograph: When you remove the barbell from the rack, place your palms on top of the bar and cross your arms in front of your chest in an X so that your arms are parallel to the floor and your elbows point forward. This method of holding the bar is easier on your wrists than using a regular overhand grip. However, make sure that the bar is secure against your body before starting your reps. If you have any doubt, don't proceed, or go back to an overhand grip. Front Squats can also be done on a Smith Machine.

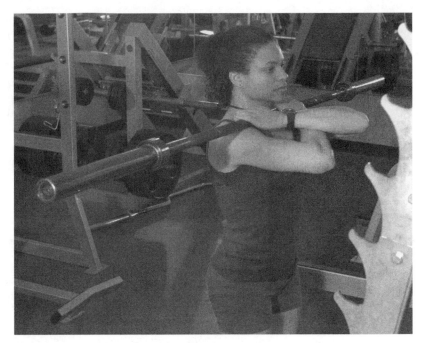

**Front Squat**

### Sissy Squat (illustrated on p. 122)

*Technique:* This is an outstanding squat exercise that uses only your body weight. Stand with your feet shoulder-width apart and your toes pointing out slightly. Hold onto a support with one hand. Then bend your knees fully, squatting to the floor. At the same time, rise up on your toes and lean your torso back at about a 45-degree angle, continuing to hold onto the support. Lower your body until your buttocks almost touch your heels, but don't go any lower than is comfortable. Feel your thigh muscles stretch. Pause at the bottom, then slowly stand up.

NOTE: Despite its name, this exercise is more difficult than it might appear. Sissy Squats can help develop extreme definition in your thighs. Some people prefer to do them between a set of dip bars because you can hold the bars on both sides for support. Experiment with the width of your stance. Some people get better results when using a narrower stance. More advanced bodybuilders often hold a barbell plate against their chest for extra resistance.

### Hack Squat

*Technique:* This exercise uses a piece of equipment similar to the Smith Machine, described above. A Hack Machine also has rails for weight to travel on, but they are angled at 45 to 60 degrees, not vertically. In addition, a Hack Machine doesn't use a barbell; instead, you place weights on a platform that moves up and down like a sled. To start, lie on your back on an inclined pad (with your head at the top) and rest your shoulders against two supports. With your feet on a platform near the floor, bend your knees fully. Grab the handles next to your head for support. Make sure you feel comfortable, then press your legs against the bottom platform, moving your torso (and the weights) along the rails. At the top, pause, then bend your knees and gradually lower your body to the starting position.

NOTE: This machine offers the same advantage as a Smith Machine: You don't have to balance a barbell on your shoulders to do a squatting motion. The tilted angle of the Hack Machine

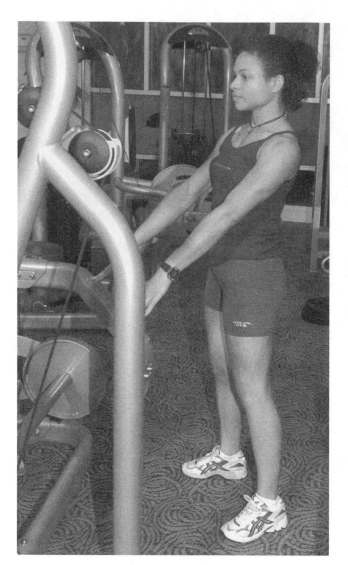
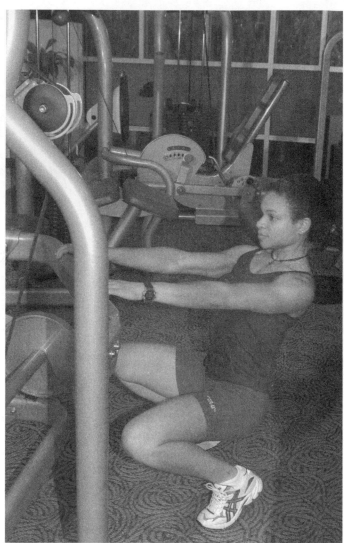

**Sissy Squat**

works your thighs in a different way than the vertical movement of the Smith Machine. When you first use a Hack Machine, have your feet shoulder-width apart and point your toes out slightly. Then try changing the positioning of your feet and toes. With each change, you'll get a slightly different result from your workout.

### Leg Press

*Technique:* This exercise uses a piece of equipment similar to a Hack Machine: It has a seat with a back and a platform at head-height attached to a weight stack. Sit on the seat and

bend your knees fully until your thighs are near your chest. Place your feet on the platform and press firmly against the platform until your legs straighten and your knees lock, raising the stack of weights. Hold, then bend your knees again and return the weight to the starting position.

NOTE: The Leg Press has an advantage over Squats because it places no stress on your lower back and you don't have to balance the weight. Your thighs do all the work of raising and lowering the weight. As with Hack Squats, you can vary the position of your feet. Some Leg Press machines, especially older ones, require you to lie on your back and push straight up on a weight platform that's directly overhead. A machine with this design isn't as comfortable to use as one that allows you to push against weights at about a 45-degree angle, and it's generally not as effective.

### Leg Extension (illustrated on p. 31)

*Technique:* This exercise uses a machine widely found in gyms. Designs vary slightly, but they typically have a seat with a back to lean against and padded rollers, attached to a weight stack, to tuck your legs under. Sit on the seat, bend your knees at a 90-degree angle, and place your shins against the two roller pads with the tops of your feet underneath the pads for stability. Grab the handles on either side of the seat for support, then raise your lower legs up in a semicircular motion until your legs are straight and can't go any higher. Pause, then return to the starting position.

NOTE: Keep the rest of your body, including your upper legs, steady as you lift with your lower legs. Don't let your back move forward or your buttocks come off the seat. You want your thighs to do all the work. Never "kick" up the weight up in a jerky manner. Likewise, don't let the weight drop without any resistance. Strive for a steady, smooth motion as you lift and lower the weight. Leg Extensions can produce outstanding definition in your thighs. As an alternative, you can lift one leg at a time, using less weight.

### Lying Leg Curl

*Technique:* This exercise is an excellent complement to Leg Extensions. Whereas extensions focus on the front of the thigh, leg curls work the back—the hamstring area. These muscles aren't as showy as the quadriceps muscles in front, but they are essential for complete thigh development. This exercise is somewhat similar to the Standing Barbell Curl for your biceps. You start by lying face down on a flat bench that has a floor-level pulley with a weight stack. Extend your knees off one end of the bench and place your ankles under two roller pads. Grab the side of the bench for support. Then raise your lower legs up and back toward your buttocks in a wide arc. During the movement, keep your upper body and thighs firmly against the bench. Stop lifting when the roller pads touch (or come close to) your buttocks. At the end of the movement, it's okay to arch your back a little and come off the bench to lift the weight a few more inches. Pause, then slowly lower the weight.

NOTE: Be sure not to "kick" up the weight at the start of the motion. Form is much more critical than using heavy weight. You want a steady, gradual movement up and down. You may find that it is difficult to use a lot of weight at first, but that's okay—many beginning bodybuilders have weak hamstrings. Instead of lying face down on the bench, you can try resting your weight on your elbows. This may keep your torso from rising off the bench. Some people with back problems find that even when done properly, Lying Leg Curls are painful. If you find them painful, don't do them. If you still choose to do this exercise, however, you can lift with one leg at a time.

### Standing Leg Curl

*Technique:* The Standing Leg Curl also works the hamstrings. It's done on the machine used for Leg Extensions, described above. Your starting position is different, however: You stand instead of sit. Stand at the end of the seat, facing the weight stack, and place your lower calves against the roller pads. Hold the machine for support, then lift or "curl" one leg at a time toward your buttocks. Raise the weight as high as you can while keeping your upper body stationary. Pause, then lower it. Reverse legs.

NOTE: To change the effect on your hamstrings, you can angle your feet in different directions. Keep your back straight until you reach the top of the motion, then arch your back slightly to lift the weight a few more inches. If you have back problems, do this exercise carefully. You may prefer to do Lying Leg Curls or Standing Leg Curls, which are similar, depending on which is more comfortable.

### Cable Kick

*Technique:* This exercise has many variations. Although it isn't performed very often, it can be extremely effective. Stand next to a machine that has a floor-level pulley. Attach a leather loop handle, or cuff (instead of a metal handle), to the end of the cable. Place the loop around your left ankle and stand facing the machine. Step back a few feet and hold onto the machine. You may want to lean forward at a 45-degree angle for added stability. Gradually, move your left leg back until you've taken up the slack in the cable.

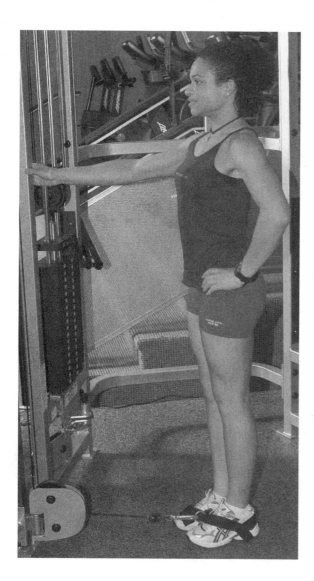
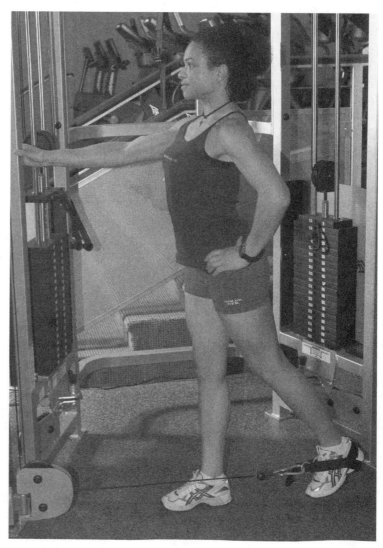

**Cable Kick**

This is the starting point. Now kick your left leg back and up, raising the weight. You'll only move your leg about 3 feet—not all the way to your buttocks. Pause when you can't lift your leg any higher, then gradually lower your leg to the starting position. After you complete your reps, reverse legs.

NOTE: The Cable Kick works your thighs but also your buttocks, making it a valuable exercise. You need firm buttocks to complement your thighs. As an alternative, you can stand on a block so that your foot doesn't hit the floor as you lower the weights.

*Variations:* We have described the movement when facing the weight stack, but the Cable Kick can be per-

formed facing in any direction. You can face away from the weight stack and raise your leg in front of your body, or you can stand with either side toward the weights and raise your leg laterally.

### Lunges

*Technique:* Lunges are somewhat similar to Squats in that you hold a barbell behind your head, resting it across the back of your shoulders. Bend your knees and get under the bar so that it's on your shoulders. Grab it with an overhand grip and with your hands slightly more than shoulder-width apart. Straighten your legs to take the bar off the rack, and step forward

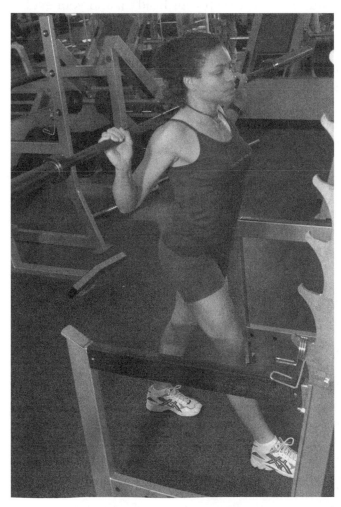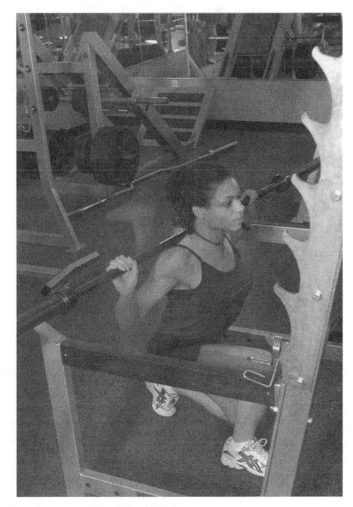

Lunges

slightly. Position your feet about shoulder-width apart. Now, instead of squatting straight down, take a big step—about 2 feet—forward with your right leg, bending it fully at the knee. This causes your torso to sink toward the floor. Your right knee will be in front of your body. At the same time, your left leg will extend behind you and be bent slightly at the knee for stability. As you lower yourself toward the floor, keep your back straight, your chest thrust out, and the barbell firmly balanced on your shoulders. Make sure your head is up and your eyes are looking forward. When your body is at the lowest point, pause, then bring your left leg forward until it's even with your right and slowly stand up. When you're standing straight, pause again to make sure you have a firm grasp on the barbell, then take another big step forward with your left leg. This time, your right leg will extend behind you. After lowering your body as far as possible, bring your right leg forward until it's even with your left and slowly stand up. Repeat this movement, alternating legs.

NOTE: Like Cable Kicks, Lunges are excellent for developing your buttocks. Make sure that you use only light weight at first; you don't want to be so worried about balancing the bar on your shoulders that you can't concentrate on the lunging motion. In the beginning, you can even do Lunges with no weight at all, just practicing the leg movement. As another alternative, you can do Lunges with a dumbbell in each hand, which removes the challenge of balancing a barbell on your shoulders. If you have knee problems, be careful about lowering yourself too far in this exercise.

### Straight-Leg Deadlift

*Technique:* This exercise is a variation of the Deadlift, described in the section on lower back exercises. You start the same way—by stepping up to a barbell that's lying on the floor—but instead of bending your knees as you grab the bar, you keep your legs straight. Your back is then parallel to the floor. Grab the barbell with an overhand grip and your hands about shoulder-width apart. Gradually raise your torso until you're standing upright with the bar in front of your thighs. Keep your arms straight throughout the exercise and maintain a very slight bend in your knees. At the top, pull your shoulders back and thrust your chest forward to stand fully erect. Pause, then bend from the waist until the barbell is only a few inches off the floor. Then lift it again for another rep. Keep your head up and your eyes looking forward to avoid straining your neck.

NOTE: Just as with the regular Dead-lift, never jerk the barbell up or drop it to the floor. Use light weight at first and add weight cautiously. You won't be able to lift nearly as much weight as with Deadlifts, because your legs aren't providing assistance. As an alternative, you can perform the Straight-Leg Deadlift with dumbbells instead of a barbell. If you use a barbell, you can stand on a platform to let you lower the weight farther. However, the extra distance may cause back pain, so be careful.

### Calves

#### Standing Calf Raise

*Technique:* This exercise is perhaps the most effective calf exercise, and it's been a standby for decades. It can be done with a barbell or with a machine.

If you use free weights, place a barbell across the back of your shoulders as you would for Squats or Lunges. (Again, it's best to take a barbell off a shoulder-height rack than to lift it off the floor.) Your hands and feet should be about shoulder-width apart. Make sure the bar is secure on your shoulders, then place the balls of your feet on a block about 2 or 3 inches high. Keep your heels on the floor. Being careful to keep your balance, rise up until your heels are higher than your toes. Feel your calf muscles stretch. When you're as high as you can go, pause, then lower yourself to the starting position with your heels on the floor. Let them touch only briefly before starting another rep.

If you use a machine, bend your knees and place your shoulders against two padded bars that resemble a yoke. Put the balls of your feet on a block,

as described above. Holding the shoulder supports with both hands, raise your body until your heels are higher than your toes. Pause, then lower yourself.

NOTE: Keep your body in one continuous line throughout the movement. Don't bend your torso to the front or rear. If you do Standing Calf Raises with a barbell, it's essential to maintain a firm grasp on the weight throughout the movement and to keep your balance. Use light weight at first until you become comfortable with the motion. As you gain experience, you can use a taller block—up to about

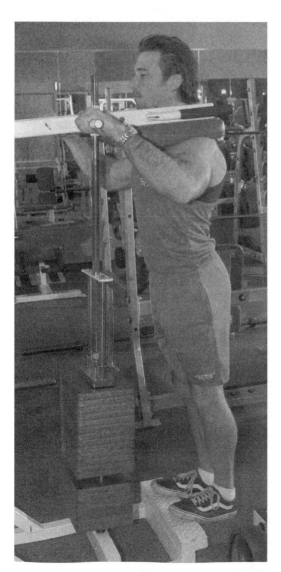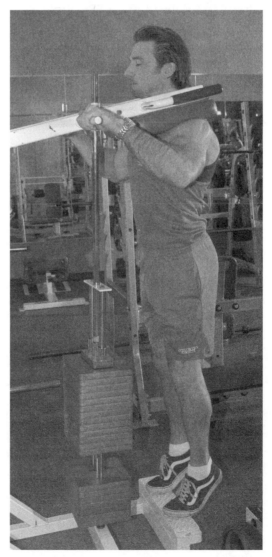

**Standing Calf Raise**

4 inches high. With a calf machine, you don't have to balance the weight on your shoulder: You simply raise your body up. If your gym doesn't have a calf machine, you can use a Hack Machine, described above for thigh work. It has twin supports for your shoulders and a sled that holds weights for resistance. Position yourself under it and straighten your legs. To do the Standing Calf Raise, rise up on the balls of your feet and then lower your heels to the starting position. Whether you use free weights or a machine, you can change the positioning of your feet or your toes for different effects. Be sure not to "bounce" up at the bottom of the motion to help you lift the weight.

*Variations:* The Standing Calf Raise has variations that you may want to try:

- You can lift with one leg at a time, instead of both together. This is particularly useful if one calf is larger than the other, because you can work more on the smaller leg until the calves are about the same size. You should measure your calves first to make sure that the size difference is real and that your eyes aren't deceiving you.
- You can use dumbbells instead of a barbell or machine. Hold a dumbbell in one hand, with your palm turned inward. With the other hand, hold onto a bar or machine for support as you raise and lower yourself.

### Seated Calf Raise

*Technique:* This exercise is identical to the Standing Calf Raise, except that you sit instead of stand. It can be done more effectively on a machine designed specifically for the Seated Calf Raise than with a barbell. Sit on the seat, with your thighs under a padded horizontal bar. Place the balls of your feet on a platform on the floor. Then raise your heels, pressing your thighs against the pads and lifting a weight stack. At the top, pause, then lower your legs until your heels are on the floor again. If you don't have access to a seated calf machine, you can place a barbell across the tops of your thighs near your knees, then lift and lower the weight. Place a towel under the bar for comfort, and hold the bar securely so that it doesn't roll back and forth.

NOTE: Keep your torso stationary and perpendicular to the floor throughout the exercise. Otherwise, you're bringing other muscles into play and reducing the benefit to your calves. Develop a smooth, rhythmic motion as you lift and lower the weight.

### Calf Raise on Leg Press Machine

*Technique:* This type of Calf Raise uses the Leg Press machine, described in the thigh section. Sit, bending your knees toward your body. Place the bottom of your feet on a platform in front of you, which may be at eye level or lower. To begin, press firmly against the platform until your legs straighten, raising the weight. Position your feet so that only the balls of your feet are on the platform, then push up so that you're working only your calf muscles. When your feet are fully extended, pause, then allow your feet to return to the starting position.

NOTE: Some Leg Press machines, usually older ones, have a vertical instead of horizontal design. That is, you lie on your back and press straight up, instead of out, on the weights. This type of machine isn't as comfortable, but you can still use it for calf raises. Follow the technique described above. As with any calf exercise, you can vary the positioning of your feet or your toes for different effects.

### Reverse Calf Raise

*Technique:* As the name implies, the Reverse Calf Raise is the opposite of

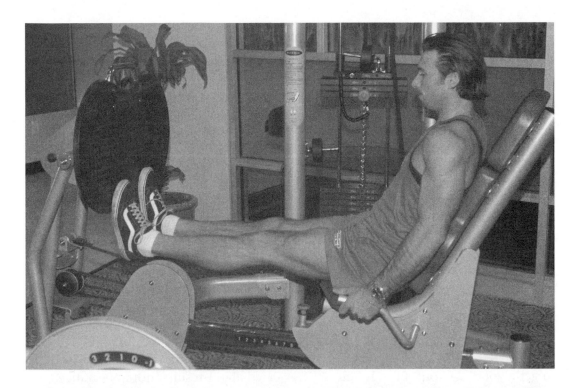

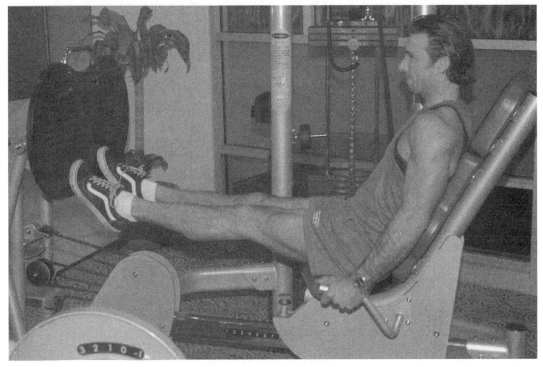

**Calf Raise on Leg Press Machine**

the standard Calf Raise. You stand with your heels (instead of the balls of your feet) on a block or platform. Make sure you are properly balanced on your heels before beginning. Without moving your heels, raise your toes toward your chest. At first you should try this movement without weight, because it can seem awkward. As you lift and lower yourself, hold onto an object for support.

NOTE: Reverse Calf Raises are good because they work the muscles at the *front* of your lower legs. Traditional calf raises focus on the rear muscles. The muscles in front aren't as prominent or showy, but they must be built up to have complete lower leg development. They can also add significantly to the overall size of your calves.

### Donkey Calf Raise

*Technique:* This exercise, which isn't done often, is identical to the Standing Calf Raise, except that you have someone sitting on your back as you go up and down. This may seem odd, and it does look a little strange, but the idea is to increase the resistance as you do calf raises. Otherwise, you may not be able to hold enough weight to get a good workout. Even if you're using a machine, it may not provide enough resistance. Having a friend sit on your back solves that problem. To start, bend your torso until it's parallel to the floor and hold onto an object for support. Place the balls of your feet on a block, then have a partner sit on your back as close to your buttocks as possible with legs hanging loosely down. Make sure the partner is secure on your back and is not causing you pain. Then do normal calf raises, raising and lowering your heels.

NOTE: You may feel somewhat strange performing this exercise, but it's a good one nonetheless. As you become more advanced, your calves may get so strong that you need more and more weight. Arnold Schwarzenegger swore by Donkey Calf Raises during his heyday in the 1970s, and there are black-and-white photos of him with *two guys* on his back. Arnold cared about results, not appearance. You'll never need to try that— you might not even be able to find two guys who *want* to sit on your back.

# 9

# Intermediate Abdominal Exercises

"Well-toned abs go hand in hand with total health and lower back integrity. There is also great psychological value to having tightly muscular abdominals."

—John Hnatyschak, former top bodybuilder

Bodybuilders throughout time have always wanted to develop their arms, chest, shoulders, and legs, but only in recent years have they devoted the same attention to their abdominal muscles, commonly called abs.

Bodybuilding contestants today know that a great set of abs is just as important as any other muscle group in winning an event. As a beginner, you shouldn't overlook your abs either. Some people have a negative image of stomach exercises: They remember doing countless sit-ups in gym class as kids—and hating it. Today, we're aware of many other ab exercises that are more effective and more enjoyable.

Most people have a real incentive to do ab exercises. After all, who doesn't want a flat, hard stomach? It's great to have broad shoulders and massive biceps, but a protruding stomach will certainly dull the impression they make. Ab exercises, done properly and faithfully, can tighten, tone, and add definition to your midsection.

Genetics comes into play in developing your abs, just as it does in working your other muscles, so that some people can achieve a rock-hard, sculpted "six-pack" relatively easily. Even if you're lacking in the gene department, though, you can still improve your midsection tremendously.

Look at today's top bodybuilders. Their ab muscles put to shame those of their predecessors of the 1950s, '60s, and even '70s. Over the years, much more importance has been attached to ab development, and bodybuilders have learned more effective ways to train these muscles. In addition, there's a much better understanding of nutrition. Diet has a huge effect on abs: If you eat too much fat, you'll never be able to achieve great definition of your abs because a layer of fat will cover the muscles.

It's a misconception that you can take several inches off your waist with ab exercises alone. This is called "spot reduction," and it doesn't work, despite the ads for some workout equipment.

If you're overweight and flabby, you have to improve your diet and do a lot of aerobic work, such as running or riding a bike. Once you shed pounds, you can tighten, firm, and flatten your stomach. The ab exercises we'll describe aren't miracle workers, and they can't produce washboard abs in a matter of days. Combined with an overall fitness plan, though, they are effective.

"I'm amazed at how many people still believe that all you have to do to get good abs are abdominal exercises," says Lee Labrada, a two-time Mr. Olympia runner-up. "You hear people say things like, 'I'm going to work off my beer belly. A hundred sit-ups a day for a month ought to do it.'

"That's the fallacy about spot reduction. The persistence of this myth is what sells needless gimmicks to the public."

Beginning bodybuilders tend to go full bore in developing their arms, chest, and shoulders, while ignoring their abs. Granted, abs aren't as visible as the upper body muscles, but they're just as important. A narrow waist and tight midsection will accentuate the development in your shoulders, chest, and arms. You can't achieve the extreme V shape necessary in body-building without a small waist.

Besides improving your appearance, well-developed abs help support your lower back during heavy lifting. Many people suffer back injuries, in part because they haven't developed their abs. Taller, heavier men sometimes have more trouble achieving outstanding definition in their abs, but that doesn't mean they shouldn't work at it.

"Years ago, contest judges didn't really expect heavyweight body-builders—those weighing over 200 pounds in contest condition—to have sharply delineated abdominal muscles," says Lee Haney, an eight-time Mr. Olympia. "The bigger men could get away with having plenty of muscle mass to complement their lofty stature. . . . Today, men competing at body weights of up to 250 pounds . . . must have total abdominal development."

Some bodybuilders make the mistake of adding mass at the expense of their abs, but it's not worth packing a few more inches onto your chest and arms if your midsection also grows. Body-building success is all about proper proportion.

"I have often seen contests in which good bodybuilders came in a few pounds overweight in order to appear bigger, but the extra weight they were carrying at the waist spoiled the effect," Arnold Schwarzenegger says. "The sport has become so com-petitive that there is no longer any such thing as a champion bodybuilder without excellent abs at almost any level of competition."

Ab exercises are intended to create shape and separation in the muscles of your midsection, but it's possible to develop your abs *too much,* so that your waistline grows instead of shrinks—you would lose the effect you were after in the first place! For this reason, most ab exercises don't involve weights. Your own body weight provides enough resistance. Contrary to what some people think, there's no need to do hundreds of repetitions on ab exercises. You can stick to 15 to 20 reps if you use proper form.

"I find that once my abs are in shape, I don't have to do too much to maintain them," says Dorian Yates, six-time Mr. Olympia winner. "Too much ab work causes thickening of the waistline."

All effective ab exercises use some type of "crunching" motion—contract-ing your abs. This can be done either by bringing your rib cage down toward your waist or by bringing your waist up toward your rib cage. In the exercises that follow, you'll see a wide variety of motions. Some exercises are per-formed on the floor, some on a flat bench, some on an incline bench, and some on machines. You need to work your abs thoroughly from a number of angles, just as you do any muscle. Some of these exercises will be more comfortable and more effective than others. There's no need to force yourself to do an exercise that doesn't feel right or that doesn't seem to be working.

## EXERCISES

### Incline Board Sit-Up

*Technique:* Lie on your back on an incline board with your head at the bottom. Hook your feet under two roller pads that are just below the top of the board; this way, you won't slide down. Clasp your hands behind your head (fingers interlocking) with your elbows pointing outward. Raise your head slightly off the bench, then roll your shoulders and upper torso toward your knees in one motion. Stop when your torso is perpendicular to the floor and your abs are still flexed. Hold, then slowly lower yourself—but stop about 8 inches from the bench. By not going all the way down on each rep, you help avoid back problems. At the lowest point, pause, then raise your torso back to perpendicular.

NOTE: Don't bring your torso so far forward that your elbows touch your knees, for the same reason that you don't lower yourself all the way: Both can cause back pain or injury. All the benefit to your abs comes in the middle part of the motion. Don't raise your torso abruptly on the first rep. Raise and lower yourself gradually and under control. To make the Incline Board Sit-Up more difficult and more effective, twist your torso slightly in either direction as you bring your torso forward. Turn a little to the left on one rep, so your right elbow points at your left knee. On the next rep, do the reverse. This way, you work the intercostal muscles at the top and sides of your abs. For variety, you can hold

a light weight behind your head to add resistance. If you find this exercise painful, skip it. There are other abdominal exercises that are just as effective.

### Roman Chair Sit-Up (illustrated on p. 134)

*Technique:* This exercise is done on a specially designed bench. A Roman chair has a seat that's about knee high (with no back) and a low horizontal bar near the floor in front of the seat. Sit upright with your legs bent toward the floor. Extend your legs slightly and place your feet under the support, pressing them up against it. Fold your arms across your chest in an X. Lean your torso back until it's almost parallel to the floor—this is the start of the movement. Now raise your torso several inches toward your knees (but well short of upright) until your abs no longer flex. Pause, then lower yourself to the starting position before raising your torso again.

NOTE: As you sit up, you should feel a "crunching" sensation in your abs. This exercise involves a very short range of motion—only a few inches. Yet it can help produce rock-hard abs. You can also twist from side to side as you do the reps. Be careful not to "bounce" at the bottom of the motion or to swing your torso up—this takes effort away from the abs. Keep your legs stable on the bench.

### Crunches (illustrated on p. 135)

*Technique:* Crunches are a very effective ab exercise with several variations. For the basic crunch, lie on the floor with a flat bench crosswise in front of you. Rest the backs of your calves and ankles on the bench, with your legs bent at a 90-degree angle. Clasp your hands behind your head (fingers interlocking), raise your head slightly off the floor, then roll your shoulders toward your knees a few inches. Don't lift your back off the floor; this can cause injury, and it

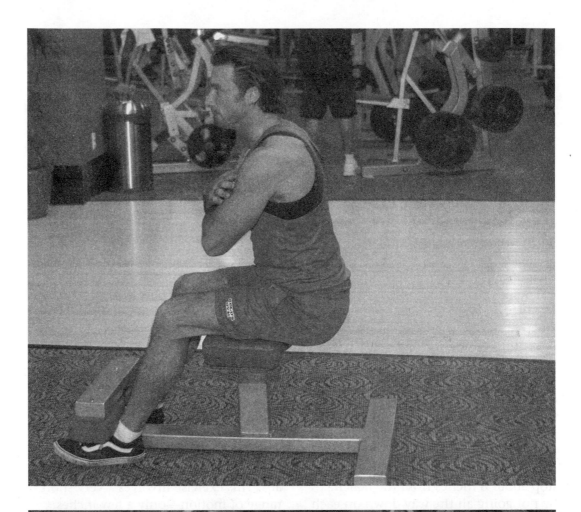

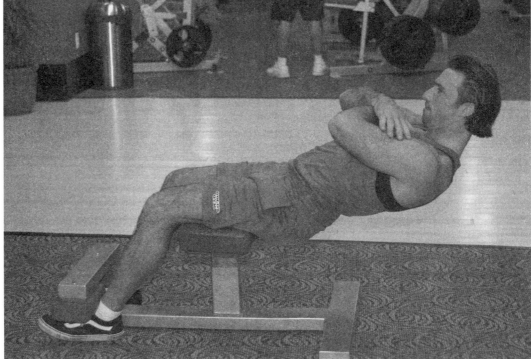

**Roman Chair Sit-Up**

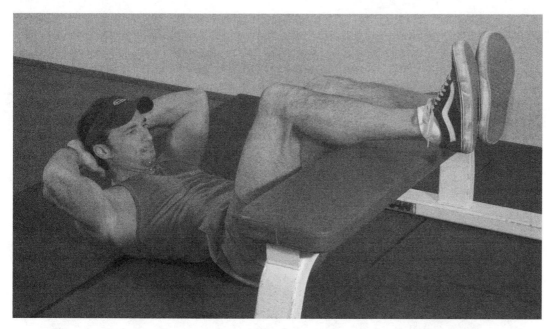

**Crunches**

doesn't benefit your abs. As you raise yourself, "crunch"—or flex—your abs.

NOTE: As alternatives, you can cross your arms across your chest instead of clasping your hands behind your head or you can twist from side to side as you sit up. Do each rep slowly and deliberately. You should be able to feel your abs contracting and strengthening. Don't thrust your shoulders forward on the way up.

### Reverse Crunch (illustrated on p. 136)

*Technique:* As the name implies, the Reverse Crunch is essentially the opposite of standard Crunches. Instead of "crunching" your torso toward your legs, you crunch your legs toward your torso. Lie on a flat bench with your head at one end. Reach back and grab the bench behind your head for support, keeping your forearms against the sides of your head. Bend your knees fully and bring your legs toward your chest as far as possible without raising your lower back off the bench—this is the starting point. Now curl your knees toward your face until they touch your elbows, which are pointing up,

so that your back is completely off the bench with your weight resting on your shoulder blades. Pause, then lower your legs until your lower back is on the bench again.

NOTE: As your knees near your elbows, you should feel the "crunch." When you lower your legs to the starting position, you'll feel a stretch. Do this movement slowly and deliberately. You should feel as if you're rolling into a ball, and then unrolling.

### Cable Crunch

*Technique:* Attach a 2-foot long rope to the end of the cable on an overhead-pulley cable machine. Kneel in front of the machine and pull both ends of the rope toward the floor to make an inverted V. Grab the big knots at each end. Position your arms so that the ends of the rope are just in front of your forehead and your elbows are close to your side. Lean forward. Now pull down on the rope with your torso, keeping your elbows close to your side and your lower body stationary. Pull downward until your head is close to the floor, your elbows are close to

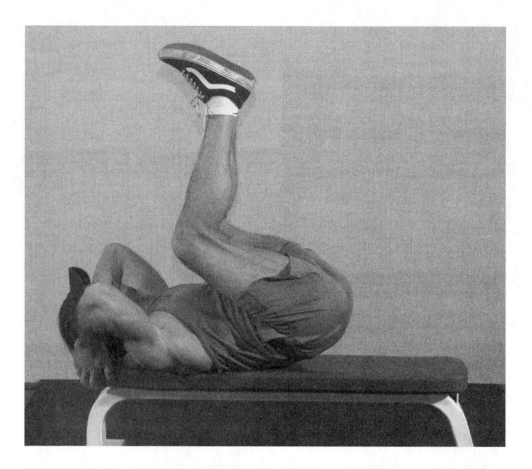

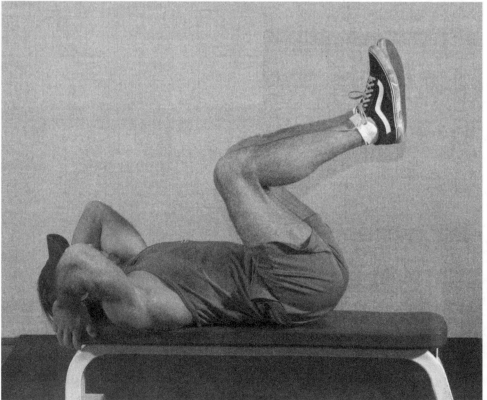

**Reverse Crunch**

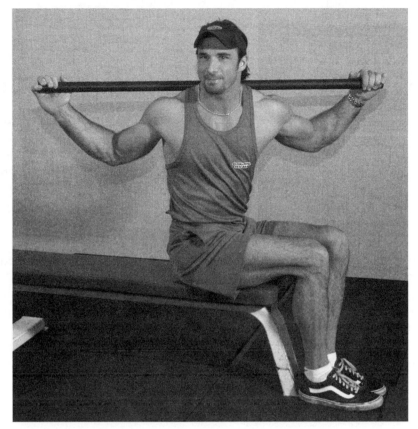

**Twists**

your knees, and your torso is parallel to the floor. Hold, then return to the starting point.

NOTE: Keep in mind that this is an ab exercise. Don't pull down on the cable with your arms. You want your abs to pull the weight down as you lower your torso.

### Machine Crunch

*Technique:* A variety of machines, some more effective than others, have been developed to work the abs. On most machines, you lie on your back on a bench, bend your knees, and place your feet under two roller pads. Then you grab two handles that are either at the sides of your chest or behind your head. This is the starting position. Now perform the crunching motion—raising your head, shoulders, and torso off the bench—until you can't go any higher. Pause, then

lower your body to the starting position.

NOTE: On some machines, you start by sitting upright and grabbing two handles behind your head. Then you crunch forward while holding the handles. Some bodybuilders dislike all ab machines because they think they only benefit from exercises using benches. Judge for yourself. Successful bodybuilding is all about learning what works for you.

### Twists

*Technique:* This exercise uses no weights—only a long bar (or broom handle). Sit on the end of a flat bench with your feet on the floor. Place the bar behind your head, resting it across the back of your shoulders, and hold it. Keeping your head still and your eyes looking forward, bend your torso to the right as far as possible. Your shoulders should rotate at about a 90-degree angle so that they're turned sideways. Hold, then rotate in the opposite direction.

NOTE: You want a slow, deliberate motion to work the abs. Be careful not to swing your torso from side to side. Keep your buttocks and thighs firmly on the bench—don't let them lift up. For variety, you can stand and perform the same movement, with your feet slightly more than shoulder-width apart. You can also bend forward from the waist so that your torso is almost parallel to the floor, then twist from side to side. As you do, keep your head down and your eyes looking at the floor in front of your feet. Do the motion under control. Twisting movements— whether standing or seated—develop the intercostal muscles at the top and sides of your abs. Twists are also an excellent warm-up exercise at the beginning of your workout because they loosen up the entire upper body. You can hold a bar with an overhand grip using your fingers or you can place your wrists and lower forearms on top of the bar to support it.

### Side Bend

*Technique:* Stand with your feet about shoulder-width apart and hold a light dumbbell in your left hand at your side. Lean your torso to the right as far as possible, bending only from the waist. Extend your right arm down toward the floor for balance. The dumbbell in your left hand will act as a counterweight to help you lower and raise your right side smoothly. After you've finished the reps, hold the dumbbell in your right hand and repeat, bending to the left.

NOTE: Be sure to use light weight and perform high reps—about 20 on each side. If you use heavy weight and do low reps (8 to 10), you'll build bulk through your waist. Side Bends should tone and tighten your midsection, not overdevelop the muscles.

### Hanging Leg Raise

*Technique:* Grab an overhead bar— the type used for Chin-Ups—with an overhand grip and with your hands shoulder-width apart. Let your body hang straight down. Bend your knees slightly and extend your legs straight out until they are parallel to the floor and even with your waist. Keep your upper body stationary so that you don't swing your legs up. When your legs are parallel, hold for a second, then lower them under control to the starting position. Keep your lower legs slightly in front of your body as you end each rep, so that your torso and legs aren't in a straight line. This helps prevent you from rocking backward, which puts stress on your lower back. If swaying remains a problem, have a partner gently hold your hips as you raise and lower your legs.

*Variations:* The Hanging Leg Raise has variations:

- Start with your legs hanging straight down, as above. As you begin to raise your legs, bend them fully at the knee and then twist both thighs to the left. On the next rep, do the same but twist both thighs to the right. Raise your thighs slightly higher than parallel to the floor. As you twist either direction, feel your abs "crunch." Keep your toes pointed slightly downward. Some people find that this variation places less stress on the lower back than the basic Hanging Leg Raise.
- Start with your legs hanging straight down, then bend your knees so that your thighs are parallel to the floor— this is the starting position. Hold this position, and then raise your knees together as high as you can toward your chest. At the same time, curl your shoulders forward. You'll

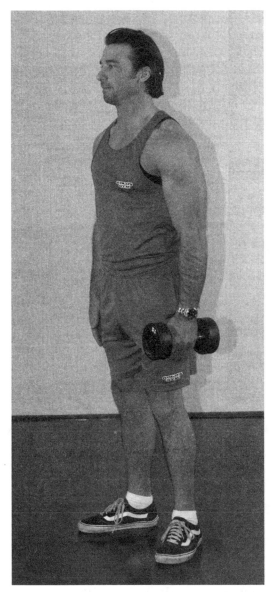
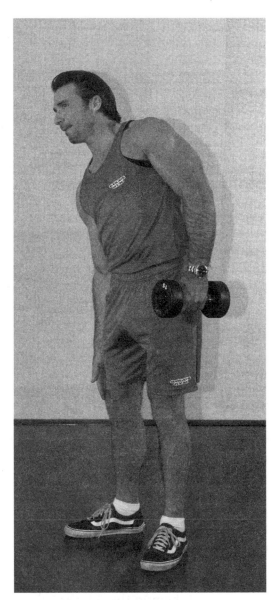

**Side Bend**

feel as if you're rolling up into a ball. Point your toes slightly downward. Pause, then lower your legs to the starting position, with your thighs parallel to the floor. If your legs are well-developed and heavy, you may have difficulty doing this variation.

### Parallel Bar Leg Raise

*Technique:* For this exercise, use a piece of equipment similar to Dip bars that has two short, parallel horizontal bars about chest high and shoulder-width apart. Place your forearms on the padded bars, with your hands in front of you, and grab the handles at the ends of the bars. Bend your knees and raise your thighs until they're parallel to the floor—this is the starting position. Pull your knees toward your chest as far as possible, round your shoulders as if rolling into a ball, and point your toes slightly downward. Feel your abs crunch. Hold, then lower your thighs back to the starting position.

NOTE: Be sure to hold your upper body steady so that you don't swing your legs up. For variety, you can raise one leg at a time from the starting point.

### Bench Leg Raise

*Technique:* The Bench Leg Raise is an effective exercise that has many variations. To start, lie on your back with your buttocks at the end of a flat bench and your legs straight out in line with your torso. Grab the end of the bench under your buttocks for support. (Alternatively, grab the bench behind your head.) Keeping your legs straight, raise them until they are just short of perpendicular to the floor. Hold, feeling your abs crunch, then lower them to the starting position.

NOTE: Keep your upper body and head flat on the bench. Do each rep slowly and deliberately. Don't raise your legs too high or your abs will relax. As you lower your legs, don't let them go below the top of the bench, because this places too much strain on your lower back. You can bend your knees slightly if that's more comfortable. Monitor your body. Some people experience back pain even when doing the Bench Leg Raise properly, and they need to choose other exercises instead.

*Variation:* After returning your legs to the starting position parallel to the floor, extend them to the sides as far as possible in a V. Pause, then bring your legs together and raise them vertically. As you return your legs to parallel to the floor, extend them horizontally again. Be sure to keep your upper body stationary.

### Incline Bench Leg Raise

*Technique:* This is the Bench Leg Raise performed on an incline bench. Place your head at the higher end. Grab the top of the bench behind your head for support, then raise your legs together until they are parallel to the floor—this is the starting position. Bend your knees slightly to reduce stress on your lower back, then gradually raise your legs to form a 45-degree angle with the bench. Pause, then lower them back to parallel.

NOTE: Notice that you raise your legs only 45 degrees, not 90 degrees, as with flat bench leg raises. Because your upper body is at an angle, your abs don't get any benefit by going higher than 45 degrees. Many incline benches are adjustable, so you can try different angles, but be sure to raise your legs vertically only—don't extend your legs sideways in a V.

*Variation:* At the starting point, with your legs together and parallel to the floor, bend your knees and bring your thighs toward your chest as far as possible. Hold them there, feeling the crunch. Then extend your legs together back to the starting point. Don't raise your legs overhead.

### Bench Kickback (illustrated on p. 142)

*Technique:* This exercise involves a much different movement, one that works your glutes more than your abs. For a well-developed midsection, you need strong, firm glutes. Kneel on top of a flat bench. Extend your arms perpendicular to the floor and grab the sides of the bench for support. Bend your legs at a 90-degree angle and place your knees on the bench with your back parallel to the floor. Your stance resembles that of a sprinter. Kick your right leg directly behind you until your foot is slightly higher than your head and your leg points up. It will travel in a semicircular, sprinting motion. Keep the rest of your body stationary and balanced on the bench. Then lower your right leg, bringing your knee forward, up to your right arm—the starting position. Repeat. After you finish the reps, repeat with your left leg.

NOTE: Keep your head up and your eyes looking forward throughout the exercise. This will help you remain steady on the bench. Do the reps slowly

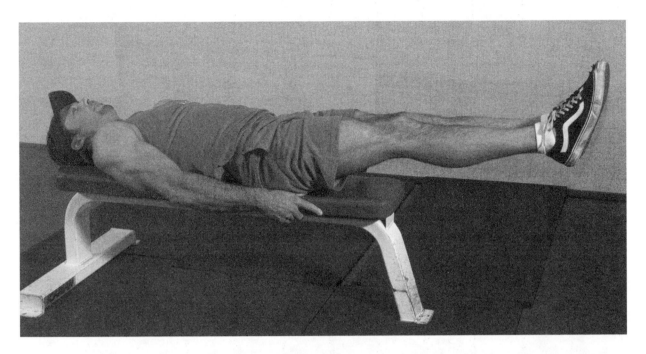

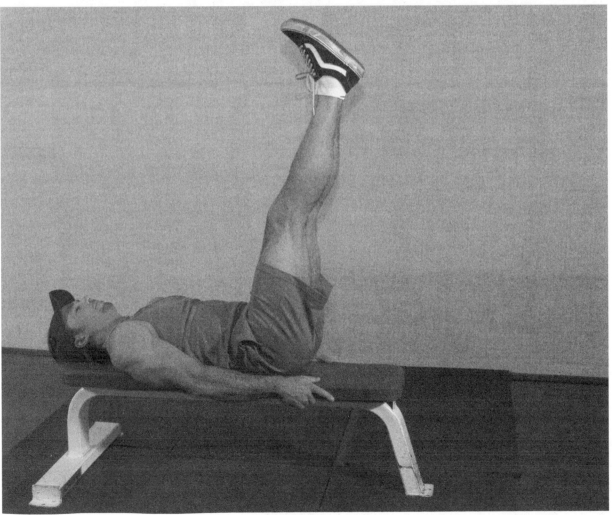

**Bench Leg Raise**

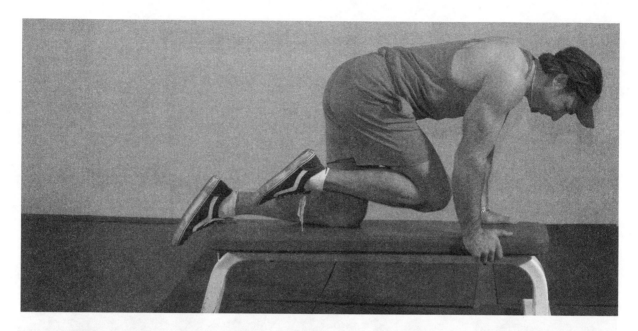

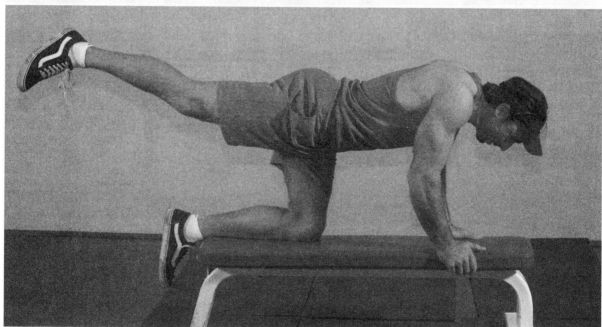

**Bench Kickback**

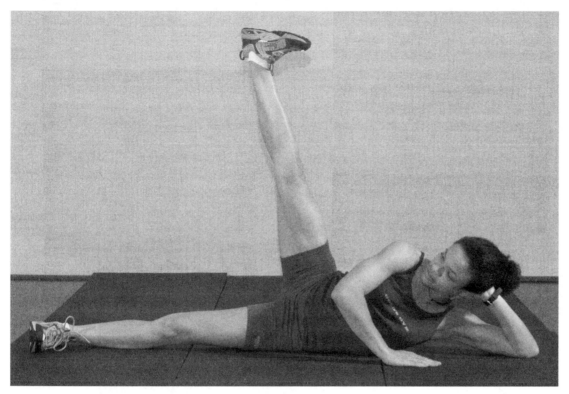

**Side Leg Raise**

and deliberately. You should quickly feel your glutes at work. This is one of the best exercises for glute development.

### Side Leg Raise

*Technique:* Lie on the floor on your left side, legs together and extended. Bend your left arm at the elbow and rest your head on your palm. Your body is now in a straight line. Keeping your right leg straight, raise it until it's perpendicular to the floor. Your foot can either point upward or be parallel to the floor. Hold, then lower your leg to the starting position, but keep it from touching your left leg. Repeat. After you finish the reps, repeat with your left leg.

NOTE: Side Leg Raises primarily work your intercostals, the muscles at the top and sides of your abs. Intercostals give your abs a complete, well-developed look. They aren't as visible as the abs themselves, but they are nonetheless important.

# 10

# The Role of Cardiovascular Exercise

"If you do aerobics all the time, your body's more efficient at burning fat. I do my main aerobic exercise on the days I don't train."

—Dorian Yates, six-time Mr. Olympia

Bodybuilders want to get big, but they can become so fixated on muscle development that they forget another important component of fitness: cardiovascular conditioning.

Cardio work, such as running or biking, builds your lung capacity and endurance. It also helps you in the gym. If you're in better cardiovascular shape, you can work out longer and harder with weights, and that's a big plus. After all, doing multiple sets with heavy weight is extremely taxing, so you need all the endurance you can get.

It's extremely shortsighted to ignore cardio, or aerobic, work. If you do, you can limit your ability to make muscle gains. We're not talking about doing hours and hours of aerobic exercise. As a general rule, about 30 minutes of cardio work three or four times a week is a good start, as long as you're disciplined about it. It's always easy to convince yourself that you need to take it easy or spend more time in the gym instead.

Many bodybuilders have the same attitude toward cardiovascular exercise that they do toward ab and leg work.

They think you can't see a healthy heart and lungs, so you're wasting your time doing it. However, aerobic exercise has another benefit besides boosting your endurance. It's far more effective at burning fat than lifting weights. If your body has less fat, you'll have greater muscle definition, so there's a direct payoff for running, biking, swimming, or any other type of cardio exercise you choose. If you make aerobic work a key part of your regimen early on, you'll likely stick with it over the long term—and reap the dividends.

Most bodybuilders do cardio exercise on the days they don't lift. This makes sense. If you try to do intense aerobics at the end of a grueling lifting session, you'll be too burned out to get results. Likewise, if you start your weight workout with strenuous cardio, you'll become fatigued, and your lifting will suffer.

However, light cardio exercise is advantageous at the start of your weightlifting sessions. Five or 10 minutes on a stationary bike, for instance, can get your heart pumping, your blood flowing, and your muscles loose so that

### ESSENTIAL AEROBICS

"For maximum results in terms of mass and cuts, bodybuilders need to do two kinds of workouts: bodybuilding workouts to build mass and aerobic workouts to burn fat....

"The ideal approach to bodybuilding involves using bodybuilding workouts to build muscle rather than to burn excess calories ... [and] doing a sufficient amount of aerobic exercise over a long enough period to burn excess fat, stimulate your metabolism and lower the fat content of your body....

"As far as diet is concerned, your goal should be to raise your caloric intake as high as possible to facilitate maximum muscle gain, while still being able to burn up excess energy using aerobic activity to avoid storing calories as fat. The result? You gain muscle and lose fat at the same time."

—from *Gold's Gym Mass Building, Training, and Nutrition System*

your body is ready to tackle an intense workout. The more you warm up, the less likely you are to strain a muscle.

A little aerobics can also be good at the end of a tough weight workout. It'll help you gradually wind down, reflect on your lifting, and make mental notes for your next workout. It's easier on your body to gradually reduce the intensity of your workout than to go full bore and then stop suddenly. In addition, cardio exercise can actually tone your muscles and help them recover from a grueling weight session.

Dorian Yates says, "I think a small amount of aerobics . . . actually helps recuperation between workouts."

What are the best forms of cardio exercise? Fortunately, you have many choices. Some people like to run; they find that jogging works their heart and lungs more in a short period than other forms of exercise. However, running can place tremendous stress on your knees, ankles, hips, and lower back, especially if you're heavy. That's because of the constant pounding of each step.

If you find that running is painful, stop. Don't try to "run through" the pain, as some people advocate. If you do, you're setting yourself up for chronic injuries that can interfere with your weight training.

If you choose to run, find a soft surface, such as grass, rather than an unforgiving concrete street. Some modern tracks have a rubberized surface that's much easier on your joints than concrete. Treadmills, which also have a softer surface, can be found in most gyms. They have the additional advantage of allowing you to adjust the speed and the angle of incline. Fast walking can be just as good as running, without as much pounding, and you can walk either on a treadmill or outdoors.

In addition, most gyms have other equipment for cardiovascular work. For example, there are stair machines that let you "climb" stairs in place. In recent years, "elliptical" machines have become popular, which simulate a running motion but offer an impact-free workout. On these machines, you stand upright and place your feet on two oval surfaces a little larger than your shoes, then you begin to "run," and the platforms move in a long, elliptical path that simulates the running motion.

If these machines aren't to your liking, you could try biking. It, too, provides excellent benefits without stress on your joints. If the weather is great, you can bike outdoors and enjoy the scenery. Of course, you can always ride a stationary bike indoors and watch TV, listen to music, or even read. Some people prefer a stationary bike even if they could ride outside.

**BODYBUILDING BIO:**
**Ronnie Coleman**

Ronnie Coleman was an intimidating cop.

Before he left the police department in Arlington, Texas, near Dallas, Officer Coleman struck fear in bad guys. Weighing close to 300 pounds, his police uniform couldn't hide his world-class muscles.

Coleman retired from the force in 2000 to devote full time to his passion—body-building. At the time, he had already won the sport's top prize, Mr. Olympia, three straight times. Since leaving law enforcement, Coleman has added three more Mr. Olympia titles.

The first time he won, he collapsed onstage in tears. He still gets emotional with each win.

"It's so overwhelming," says Coleman, who is 5'11" and competes at about 260 pounds. "It's almost better than winning the lottery because you worked for it. It's like something you want all your life, but you never thought it would happen, and all of a sudden it did."

Coleman, a former football player at Grambling State University, has a web site called *BigRonnieColeman.com.* How appropriate.

He has no intention of giving up his Mr. Olympia crown any time soon.

"I'm always challenging myself," says Coleman, 39. "I'm good at challenging myself."

Swimming is another excellent aerobic exercise. It's very demanding, and it can produce excellent results in a short amount of time, particularly if you aren't accustomed to swimming. If you haven't been swimming in a while, it may take some time to get in the groove. As you can imagine, swimming is easy on the joints. It can also be enjoyable and relaxing.

Even if you don't like to swim, you can still get a good workout in the pool by running. That may sound odd, but running in 3 or 4 feet of water provides excellent resistance and gives you a great low-impact workout. You'll be surprised at how difficult it is—you certainly won't make great time. However, your heart, lungs, and leg muscles will definitely feel the results.

Running, biking, and swimming are the most common forms of cardio exercise, but there are many more. Hiking, jumping rope, playing tennis, softball, or golf (if you walk rather than ride in a golf cart) all provide good cardio benefits. There may be other activities you enjoy that provide a good aerobic workout.

Most top bodybuilders do cardio work year-round, although some may do less during the "off season" when they're not preparing for a competition. During this time, they're usually trying to gain muscle mass, but they still want to keep their heart and lungs in good shape. In the weeks leading up to a contest, bodybuilders normally increase their aerobic exercise significantly in order to get rid of fat and improve their muscle definition.

We should also mention that it's possible to do too much cardio work. Particularly when you're in intense training, you shouldn't do lengthy, demanding aerobics—such as running long distances on a regular basis—because if you do, you'll tax your body too much. Weight training requires tremendous stamina and strength, and if your body is weak from miles of running, you won't get the full benefit in the gym. Remember—your goal is to become a bodybuilder, not a marathon runner. A cardio program should always complement your weight training, not detract from it.

Excessive cardio work can also make it difficult to retain muscle mass. If you are thin by nature, you may already have trouble gaining quality weight. If you add in too much cardio, you can sweat off your muscle as well as your fat. Be smart, and pay attention to your progress.

Everyone, no matter how thin, needs to do some aerobics in order to strengthen the cardiovascular system and build endurance. Bodybuilders who have a tendency to get too heavy may always need to do more aerobics than thinner people. Everyone is different. Success in bodybuilding depends on customizing both your weight training and your aerobics program for your physique.

# 11

# Mental Aspects of Bodybuilding

"Your mind must be in gear or all the training and nutrition
in the world won't get you anywhere."

—Lee Haney, eight-time Mr. Olympia

Your mind is a powerful tool.

In recent years, athletes in all sports have learned the value of mental preparation in order to perform their best. Bodybuilding is certainly no different. Learning to harness the power of your mind can assist you in achieving both short-term and long-term goals.

Many professional athletes use sport psychologists to help them gain a mental edge. You may not be able to afford a sport psychologist, but you can apply some of the methods they teach to achieve better results.

"Correct mental programming is essential to success in gaining humongous muscle mass and becoming a champion," says Lee Haney. "Your mental approach to bodybuilding first primes the pump and then keeps the water flowing."

You can even employ mental strength to get in the gym door and start your workout. There's always an excuse for not training:

*I don't have time.*

*I'm too tired.*

*It won't hurt to miss a workout.*

Visualization is one of the elements that sport psychologists teach. You can train yourself to "see" what you desire. In the scenario above, you could visualize yourself completing a strenuous set and imagine the satisfaction that follows. Or you could see yourself finishing your entire workout, admiring your pump, and feeling good about your progress.

Visualization can help you overcome the need to fulfill an immediate desire—in the above case, taking it easy—and achieve your true goal. Once you can imagine yourself attaining success, it's easier to overcome the obstacles that stand in your way. Soon you may discover a newfound enthusiasm for working out.

"Bodybuilders who have to force themselves to go to the gym and work out will never achieve the kind of success possible for those who can't wait to hit the gym and start pumping iron," Arnold Schwarzenegger says. "Training with this kind of enthusiasm is vital.

"The hours I spent in the gym were the high point of my day. I liked the

## YOUR STATE OF MIND

"Serious bodybuilders, committed to muscular size, ripped definition, and symmetrical enhancement, must include mental training in their bodybuilding program. Think of sports psychology as another component of training—a set of tools designed to make the best athlete possible. . . .

"You must treat mental training the same way you treat your physical training, nutritional regimen, and sleep habits. Would you enter a bodybuilding contest without working out in the gym months earlier? Could you have developed that ripped physique by adhering to a high-fat, low-protein diet? . . .

"You can develop mental skills by practicing them in a diligent and consistent manner, just as you lift weights, eat soundly, get enough rest, and take nutritional supplements. For mental skills to be effective, you must practice them every day."

—from *Mind & Muscle: Psych Up, Build Up*

way training felt, the pump I would get during my workout, and the relaxed sensation of near exhaustion that came afterward."

Your mind and body can't be separated—you can't develop your body to its fullest without enlisting the power of your mind. Schwarzenegger was one of the first bodybuilders who became known for using mental preparation to motivate himself as well as to intimidate his opponents. He was a master at "psyching out" competitors before major events.

The classic documentary *Pumping Iron* follows Arnold and several other contestants as they prepared for the 1975 Mr. Olympia competition. Arnold used his mental strength—as well as some manipulation—to make others doubt themselves on the brink of the

biggest contest of their lives. "I can make people lose," he boasted.

Some people might criticize this type of mental intimidation, but Arnold never had a problem with it. "There is always a psychological element in any sports competition," he writes in *The New Encyclopedia of Bodybuilding*. "Athletic performance at the highest levels requires a tremendous degree of self-confidence and concentration, and anything that interferes with either will seriously threaten the athlete's chances of winning.

"Nobody is immune to being psyched out. In fact, I have to admit that I've been on the receiving end of this treatment as well as dishing it out."

Most top bodybuilders, however, use psychological methods more to motivate themselves than to derail others. Unless you concentrate on your own development, you'll have no chance of defeating others—even if you're a master at manipulation.

Champion bodybuilders use mental strength to help them stick to their training schedule as well as to work out with fierce intensity. The role of intensity cannot be overstated. You can spend hours and hours in the gym, but if you aren't giving it everything you have—pushing yourself harder and harder—you're almost wasting your time. You can use visualization to create an intensity you didn't know you had.

"You won't make optimum progress toward a truly massive physique until you have a high level of mental concentration throughout each workout," says Mike Matarazzo, a top bodybuilder. "If you can concentrate fully on the working muscle, you'll be able to feel it quite intensely as it goes through its paces in a particular bodybuilding movement."

As you progress in bodybuilding, you'll invariably suffer setbacks. It might be an injury, an illness, or a commitment that gets in the way of training. When this happens, you need the mental strength to get back on track in pursuing your goals.

A few missed workouts won't doom you—unless you give in and become discouraged. That's the power of the mind. It can be your best friend or your worst enemy. Don't be like so many people who vow to get in shape but fail to follow through.

Remind yourself, over and over if necessary, that success in bodybuilding is much more a marathon than a sprint. Most likely, you won't make steady, predictable gains. You'll probably add size and definition in unpredictable spurts. You may go months without seeing any significant improvement. Just remember that if you follow your training schedule, perhaps making a few changes in your regimen, big gains are probably right around the corner. Mental strength gives you the dedication to press on when there's not an immediate payoff.

"To get really massive, you have to see yourself as being really massive," says Lee Haney. "Visualization is an exciting and effective method of programming your subconscious mind to assist it in bringing you bodybuilding success."

Champion bodybuilders aren't necessarily the ones with the greatest natural potential, but they're usually the toughest mentally. They have faced the same setbacks and hard times as other competitors, but they remain focused on their goals and they don't give up. Mental strength might seem intangible, but it's very real.

It can help you overcome failure—big or small. If you enter a bodybuilding contest and don't do as well as you had hoped, it doesn't mean that you'll never succeed. The resulting disappointment can be a motivator to train harder and smarter.

Mental strength also comes into play in your diet. As we've said, what you eat has a huge bearing on your physique. If you constantly consume junk food, your body will show it. Discipline yourself to eat right,

### YOU DON'T HAVE TO BE TALL

Height is not a requirement to be an accomplished bodybuilder.

Some of the top competitors in the history of the sport have been well under 6 feet tall.

Lee Labrada, who is 5'6", finished second in the prestigious Mr. Olympia contest in 1989 and 1990.

"A champion doesn't have to have big arms and a big chest," says Labrada, who competed at 180 pounds. "He's developed proportionately all over."

Lee regularly found himself onstage with 250-pound competitors. Yet he usually defeated them.

"I know I can't fight fire with fire, so my approach is to be the finest, the most complete, the most finished physique up there," says Labrada, 43.

He isn't the shortest person to reach the pinnacle of bodybuilding, however. Lee Priest, one of today's top competitors, is only 5'4". He's much more massive than Labrada, weighing 220 pounds in contest shape.

"How can anyone pack so much beef onto such a small frame?" a bodybuilding writer once commented.

Priest became interested in bodybuilding even before he reached puberty. By age 13, he had won three bodybuilding contests. At 17, he competed in Mr. Universe, the world's top amateur event.

"I think I got my genetics from my mother," says Lee, 31. "She took up bodybuilding at age 38 and won the state title after only eight months of training."

Shawn Ray, who stands only 5'7", was runner-up in the Mr. Olympia contest in 1994 and 1996. He's had top-five finishes in virtually every major competition around the world. It's tough to find any flaws in Shawn's physique, but he sees room for improvement.

"My bodybuilding philosophy is that you're never good enough," says Ray, 38. "Nobody is perfect. When I look in the mirror, I can see what's good about my physique, but I can see my weak points as well."

**WORDS TO TRAIN BY**

"Make the commitment and stick to it."

—Lee Priest, top bodybuilder

as tempting as it may be at times to do otherwise. Stay focused on your goals. Is that donut or cheeseburger really worth the effect it will have?

Some people use positive self-talk— also called affirmations—for motivation. Examples are "I can do this!" or "I'm the best!" You can make these statements to yourself or yell them out loud.

Athletes sometimes turn to meditation to overcome negative thoughts and focus on success. They may head to a quiet place, close their eyes, and concentrate on their goals, blocking out everything else. They might practice visualization, "seeing" themselves performing perfectly, even accepting the champion's prize.

Just as our bodies don't all perform the same way, neither do our minds. You might give yourself a pep talk that would seem corny to someone else, but if it motivates you, that's all that matters.

The mind, it's been said, is a muscle. Use it, and it will grow stronger.

"I'm the best bodybuilder in the sport," Arnold Schwarzenegger once said, "because my mind is stronger and better disciplined than others'."

# 12

# Preparing for Contests

*"I've always been a confident, outgoing person. I'm very comfortable onstage—something of a showoff—so posing in front of a big audience is easy for me."*

—Kevin Levrone, top bodybuilder

Bodybuilders share a desire to develop large, impressive physiques.

Beyond that, however, they set different goals. For most, the payoff for serious weight training is a stronger, more attractive body. Perhaps they want to prove to themselves—or to others—that they have the willpower and the discipline to reshape their physique.

A small percentage of people who turn to bodybuilding intend to enter bodybuilding contests. Arnold Schwarzenegger is a classic example. He got hooked on bodybuilding as soon as he began weight lifting, and he knew immediately that he wanted to compete. In contrast, other top bodybuilders have drifted toward competition years after they began weight training.

You certainly don't have to enter contests to be considered a bodybuilder. Anyone who faithfully develops and shapes his or her physique with weights can be called a bodybuilder. One of the sport's appeals is that you can enjoy it at all levels—from beginner all the way up to the professional ranks.

People on both ends of the spectrum share the same love of lifting weights and improving their bodies. For them, bodybuilding is a very personal endeavor. Unlike team sports, you alone dictate your goals and control your results.

If you think you'd like to enter bodybuilding contests, however, you need to know what to expect and how to prepare properly. That's the purpose of this chapter. You'll learn how to train for an event and how to do your best once you get there.

Before you decide whether to compete, you need to realize that it takes extreme commitment and dedication to be a serious contender. Just like you wouldn't decide to enter a marathon just a few weeks before the race, you can't decide that you want to compete in a bodybuilding contest just a few weeks before it is held. You must lay the foundation months, even years, in advance of a bodybuilding competition—with systematic and rigorous training.

If you've begun to develop a respectable physique, you should be able to assess whether you have the potential to compete. Genetics, which plays a huge role in bodybuilding, may be the determining factor. You might train for years and eat right, but still not have the body to enter a contest. That's okay—most people don't. Yet they can still enjoy bodybuilding.

Besides analyzing your genetic potential, you need to look at your commitments and responsibilities. If your career and home life are so demanding that you can't stick to a training regimen, you can't be a serious competitor. Again, that's fine. You can enjoy bodybuilding to the degree that it suits your lifestyle.

Once you've decided that you have the potential and you know that you have the time to train for a contest, you need to thoroughly evaluate your physique. It's best to enlist the help of an experienced bodybuilder for this. Even top competitors have weaknesses in their physique. What are yours? Once you find out, you'll be able to develop an effective training regimen.

In previous chapters, we've described numerous weightlifting exercises that cover all your muscle groups. Once you've determined your body's main weaknesses, you can pick and choose from the various exercises to develop a regimen that suits your own physique. You may do only three or four exercises for one body area if it's well developed, while you might do six or seven for another if it's lagging in development. Over time, you'll learn to evaluate your progress and make adjustments to your regimen.

It's a good idea to start by weighing yourself, because although weight is only one indicator of fitness, it's an important one. Measure your key body areas—chest, shoulders, arms, legs, and waist. Finally, have someone take photos of you in relaxed and flexed poses.

Now you have a comprehensive baseline of your physique as you begin intense training. You'll be able to set realistic goals for your development and measure yourself periodically as the event approaches.

The goal in preparing for a bodybuilding event is to peak at the right time. You want your physique to be its absolute best on the day of the contest—not a week before, not a week after. As you can imagine, timing your preparation to coincide perfectly with the contest is tricky.

Even the world's best bodybuilders sometimes miss the mark. Don't be surprised if it takes several contests to learn exactly how to organize your training so that you arrive in peak condition. Very few people place high, much less win, in their first contest. Each time you have a disappointing finish, you can gain valuable experience to help you for the next contest.

Between contests, it's normal to gain some weight and lose some definition. While you can't stay in peak form all year long—physically or mentally—make sure that you don't abandon training altogether. If you get woefully out of shape, it's much harder to whip yourself into contest condition, no matter how much time you allow.

Even though you should lift weights year-round, you won't continue to train with all-out intensity. Between contests, you'll abide by a more general workout plan and do fewer sets. Twelve to 16 weeks before a competition, you need to assess your condition and develop a detailed regimen to help you achieve your goal.

This is also the time to become more disciplined about your eating. Your pre-contest planning must include your diet and, hopefully, you won't have abandoned good eating habits altogether.

Competitive bodybuilding involves elements that people often don't consider: learning posing techniques, getting a tan, shaving your body, applying oil to highlight your muscles, and even picking out trunks that complement your physique. The many people who enjoy bodybuilding but who have no interest whatsoever in these issues shouldn't consider entering a competition. Even such seemingly small details can determine the outcome of a bodybuilding contest.

## POSING

Proper posing is critical in bodybuilding contests. You may have the best physique in the field, but if you don't know how to show it off, you won't win.

How do you feel about posing onstage in a pair of skimpy shorts, under bright lights and the scrutiny of judges? If this doesn't appeal to you, there's no use in training for a contest. Many people love the sensation of lifting weights and the satisfaction of sculpting an impressive physique, but they would be incredibly self-conscious about being onstage. People who enter bodybuilding contests must enjoy being onstage and having people stare at their bodies.

Training in the gym is one skill. Posing is an entirely different skill. Just as with lifting, there are right ways and wrong ways to pose. It's not as simple as flexing your biceps and making it as big as you can.

Bodybuilding contests have certain mandatory poses, just like figure skating competitions have compulsory elements. You must master these poses to score well. Posing is an art form that involves timing, positioning onstage, and body control.

It's also extremely strenuous. During competition, you may have to hold a pose for a minute or more. If you're not prepared, your muscles can shake or

> **WORDS TO TRAIN BY**
>
> "In preparation for a contest, I practice my posing for up to one hour at a time four or five days a week. This is increased to one hour per day over the last two weeks before a show. There's no other way for me to get it right."
>
> —Marjo Selin, top female bodybuilder

cramp. Posing may appear effortless, but it's not. "Contest posing is exhausting," says Dave Draper, a former Mr. Universe. "It's emotionally and often physically harder than the workouts that led up to posing."

In addition to mandatory poses, contestants are allowed to develop poses that highlight their strengths, as well as others that would perhaps hide their weaknesses. These vary widely, depending on a contestant's height, weight, and build.

"If you copy someone else's posing style, that's exactly what it will look like," said Cory Everson, a six-time Ms. Olympia winner. "The judges will see you as a follower, not a leader."

Whether you're doing a mandatory pose or a unique pose, your facial expression is important. You need to leave that pained, snarling look in the gym. What you want people to notice is your physique, not your face.

Arnold Schwarzenegger says, "When you are onstage, you are not only an athlete, but a performer as well."

## TANNING, OIL, AND POSING TRUNKS

Contest judges are evaluating your entire presentation. Besides posing, this includes your complexion and clothing. Here again, these may seem like silly, insignificant issues to some, but—like it or not—they're an integral part of competition. Consideration of these aspects of a bodybuilder's presentation is another opportunity to decide whether you really want to enter a bodybuilding contest.

Why is a good tan important? Because the bright lights onstage wash out a contestant with fair skin. To give yourself a fair chance, you need a tan. These days, however, we all know about the danger of spending too much time in the sun. Overexposure can cause your skin to wrinkle and age and may put you at higher risk of developing skin cancer.

To protect yourself, you must use sunscreen and limit your time outdoors. As a result, you need to start working on your tan months before a competition. Don't try to get a deep, dark tan the week of an event. You'll probably wind up beet red and burned.

Fair-skinned bodybuilders aren't the only ones who need to worry about getting a tan. "Tanning is not just for fair-skinned bodybuilders," Schwarzenegger says. "Most darker-skinned bodybuilders, like African-Americans or Latinos, find that spending some time tanning changes the skin texture and depth of tone and adds to their appearance onstage."

What about tanning booths and tanning creams? Both are okay if used in moderation. Tanning beds can be safer than direct exposure to the sun, but sunlamp rays can burn and damage your skin too.

Today's tanning lotions are far superior to those of the past, which often had the unfortunate effect of turning your skin orange. Modern creams and lotions can help you get a rich tan without the time and danger associated with long periods out in the sun or in a tanning booth, but it's a mistake to try to get your *entire* tan out of a bottle. The result probably won't

look natural. Instead, you should develop a moderate tan and then enhance it with a cream or lotion.

Onstage, even a good tan and proper posing aren't enough. To make your muscles more prominent to the judges and the audience, you must apply posing oil before you go onstage. The thought of this may not thrill you, but again, it's part of the package. Before you can apply oil, however, you've got to shave down.

Few people, at least initially, are keen about shaving all the hair off their chest, arms, and legs, but face it—hair masks the detail and definition of your muscles. Shaving and applying posing oil go hand in hand, and they serve the same purpose—to show off your muscles and give you a better chance of winning.

Don't shave for the first time the night before a contest. You're likely to cut or irritate your skin. In addition, you'll experience a psychological effect when you suddenly lose all your body hair—you'll probably feel smaller, weaker. Give yourself time to get used to the bald body look.

When you're ready to shed your hair, you can lather up and shave, as you would your face. Alternatively, you can apply hair-removal creams. These are fairly effective, but don't use them at the last minute. They, too, can irritate your skin and give you a coarse look.

Now that you've gotten rid of your body hair, it's time to put on the oil. Keep in mind, though, that too much is just as bad as too little. Beginners often slosh on posing oil indiscriminately. This makes them look shiny, and it causes light to reflect off them as if they were a mirror, which is very distracting to judges.

Oil should be applied in thin coats well before you go onstage. That way it can soak into your skin instead of staying on the surface. Once the oil is absorbed, you can add a second or even a third coat. Just don't overdo it. And don't apply a coat mere seconds before you walk onstage. It leaves a bad impression to be dripping oil. Bodybuilders use a host of different oils, from vegetable oil to olive oil. Experiment to find out what works best for you.

Besides getting a good tan and learning to use posing oil, you need to consider one other onstage detail: your shorts. There are a myriad of colors, styles, and fabrics to consider. As fashion experts will tell you, certain clothes look great on some people but terrible on others, and the same is true for posing trunks. You should consult a person who has some knowledge and experience in this area, because the wrong trunks can be as distracting to judges as too much oil.

Today, most competitors wear the briefest of shorts—essentially bikini briefs. The objective is to reveal your muscles as much as possible. Get used to wearing these shorts well before you go onstage. Just as when you shave your body hair for the first time, you're likely to feel naked and self-conscious in posing trunks at first.

## DIET AND WEIGHT LOSS

Bodybuilding contestants usually gain weight between contests to increase their muscle mass. Then as an event nears, they steadily lose weight so that their muscles will be more defined and "cut." Typically, top competitors begin a pre-contest diet 12 to 16 weeks before an event. This gives them enough time to lose up to 25 pounds— or even more, if necessary. Of course, it's best not to gain this much weight in the first place.

Once again, timing is critical. You need to start losing weight early enough to get in tiptop shape by the day of the event. Too often, contestants appear doughy and smooth because they haven't dropped enough weight. However, it's also possible to lose so much weight that you look weak and dehydrated onstage.

It takes experience to know how much to cut your calories before a contest so that you look your best in competition. By the time you begin preparing for competition, you should already understand your body's metabolism, that is, how easily your body burns calories. Once you understand your metabolism, you can more accurately plan your diet. It's unlikely that you'll diet perfectly for your first contest. There's a learning curve, just as there is with all aspects of preparation. After a few contests, though, you should be able to chart out an eating plan that gets you in lean shape just in time.

Your preparation should address not only lifting and eating but also aerobic exercise. Normally, bodybuilders increase the amount and intensity of cardio work leading up to an event. The reason is simple. They want to burn off as much fat as possible so that their muscles show more prominently. You have to be careful, though, because if you do too much aerobic exercise, you can lose muscle tissue as well as fat. Then you've undermined all your efforts to build mass.

Some bodybuilders make the mistake of using diuretics before an event so they can lose water weight, figuring that excess water detracts from their definition. Diuretics, however, can be extremely dangerous, even fatal. Your body needs an adequate amount of water for proper functioning, and muscles are made up primarily of water. If you extract water from your body with diuretics, you decrease your muscle size. Today, major bodybuilding contests test for diuretic use, just as they do for illegal drugs. Don't be tempted to break the rules and endanger your life.

Consider the tragic story of Mohammad Benaziza. After winning the 1992 Belgium Grand Prix bodybuilding contest, he dropped dead only hours later. It's believed that he died because of an electrolyte imbalance brought on by diuretic use. "Momo just froze," says bodybuilder Mike Matarazzo. "Guys who were there said he was like a piece of iron when he died."

## LAST-MINUTE WORKOUTS

Most bodybuilding contestants do some lifting and stretching immediately before going onstage. The idea is to pump up your muscles, even a little, to give yourself an edge.

You should do exercises that require no weights, such as Dips and Chin-Ups, or exercises with only light weight and high reps. Be careful not to work out so much that you become fatigued. Keep in mind that posing for long periods onstage can be exhausting, and the pressure of competition adds to your fatigue. Last-minute lifting can also pump up your muscles *too much* so that they lose critical definition.

Backstage before an event, some contestants work out together, while

---

**START EARLY**

"We have seen many bodybuilders drop more than seven pounds during a one-week period and continue to do this for several weeks. This is not dieting. It's a desperation method. It means the bodybuilder waited far too long to get serious.

"Starting late in contest preparation is the number one reason why bodybuilders fail to achieve their peaks."

—from *Sliced: State-of-the-Art Nutrition for Building Lean Body Mass*

---

others find a secluded place. There's psychological strategy at work. Some bodybuilders think it gives them an advantage to hide their physiques until they go onstage. They hope to shock opponents with their massiveness. Others, however, think it's to their advantage to show off their physiques backstage in order to demonstrate their confidence.

"Psyching out your opponents, or gamesmanship, is common to all sports," Schwarzenegger says. "None of this is cheating. Cheating is when you break the rules, not when you take advantage of an opponent's psychological weakness."

# BIBLIOGRAPHY

Connors, Edward, Peter Grymkowski, Tim Kimber, and Michael J. B. McCormick. *Building Bulk*. Chicago: NTC/Contemporary Publishing Group, 1999.

Connors, Edward, Peter Grymkowski, Tim Kimber, and Michael J. B. McCormick. *Total Torso Training*. Chicago: NTC/Contemporary Publishing Group, 2000.

Connors, Edward, Peter Grymkowski, Tim Kimber, and Bill Reynolds. *Gold's Gym Mass Building, Training, and Nutrition System*. Chicago: NTC/Contemporary Publishing Group, 1992.

Connors, Edward, Michael J. B. McCormick, Peter Grymkowski, and Tim Kimber. *The Gold's Gym Encyclopedia of Bodybuilding*. Chicago: NTC/Contemporary Publishing Group, 1996.

*Dallas Morning News*. Dallas, Tex.: October 3, 1999; May 10, 2001; and October 31, 2001.

Hatfield, Frederick C. *Hardcore Bodybuilding: A Scientific Approach*. Chicago: NTC/Contemporary Publishing Group, 1993.

Reynolds, Bill, and Negrita Jayde. *Sliced: State-of-the-Art Nutrition for Building Lean Body Mass*. Chicago: NTC/Contemporary Publishing Group, 1991.

Schwarzenegger, Arnold, with Bill Dobbins. *The New Encyclopedia of Modern Bodybuilding*. New York: Fireside/Simon & Schuster, Inc., 1999.

Schwarzenegger, Arnold, with Douglas Kent Hall. *Arnold: Arnold's Own Story*. New York: Fireside/Simon & Schuster, Inc., 1977.

Sisco, Peter. *Ironman's Ultimate Bodybuilding Encyclopedia*. Chicago: NTC/Contemporary Publishing Group, 1999.

Sisco, Peter. *Ironman's Ultimate Guide to Building Muscle Mass*. Chicago: NTC/Contemporary Publishing Group, 2000.

Thorne, Gerard, and Phil Embleton. *Encyclopedia of Bodybuilding*. Mississauga, Ontario, Canada: MuscleMag International, 1997.

Thorne, Gerard, and Phil Embleton. *Explosive Growth! Everything You Ever Wanted to Know about Building Muscle*. Mississauga, Ontario, Canada: MuscleMag International, 2000.

Thorne, Gerard, and Phil Embleton. *Muscle Quest: Training Secrets of the Superstars*, Mississauga, Ontario, Canada: MuscleMag International, 2000.

Weider, Joe, with Bill Reynolds. *Joe Weider's Ultimate Bodybuilding*. Chicago: NTC/Contemporary Publishing Group, 1989.

Whitmarsh, Blair. *Mind & Muscle*. Champaign, Ill.: Human Kinetics, 2001.

Wolff, Robert. *Bodybuilding 101*. Chicago: McGraw-Hill/Contemporary Books, 1999.

## THE STORY OF GOLD'S GYM

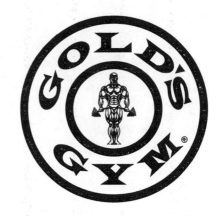

Gold's Gym has been the authority on fitness since 1965 dating back to the original Gold's Gym in Venice, California. It was the place for serious fitness. Gold's Gym quickly became known as "The Mecca of Bodybuilding." In 1977, Gold's Gym received international attention when it was featured in the movie *Pumping Iron* that starred Arnold Schwarzenegger and Lou Ferrigno. From that first gym in Venice, Gold's Gym has become the largest co-ed gym chain in the world with over 550 facilities in 43 states and 25 countries.

Today, Gold's Gym has expanded its fitness profile to offer all of the latest equipment and services, including group exercise, personal training, cardiovascular equipment, group spin, pilates and yoga, while maintaining its core weight lifting tradition. With nearly 3 million members world wide, Gold's Gym continues to change lives by helping people achieve their individual potential. For more information about Gold's Gym, please visit www.goldsgym.com or call 1-800-99-GOLDS.

*Gold's Gym has the classes you want, the equipment you need and the trainers to help you get the results you're looking for!*

The Latest Equipment • Certified Personal Training • Nutrition Counseling • Extensive Cardio • Women's Only Areas • Childcare
**Plus Hundreds of Group Exercise Classes including:** Group Spin • Yoga • Pilates • Kickboxing • Step • Stretch and More!

# FREE (14) DAY MEMBERSHIP

First time visitors only. Must be over 18 with valid ID. Must be local resident. Not redeemable for cash. Participating Gold's Gyms only. Other restrictions may apply. Amenities vary by location. ©2004 Gold's Gym International, Inc.

# Log on to www.goldsgym.com/bookoffer or call 1-800-99-GOLDS to get your free pass today!